SOUS VIDE
Gourmet Cookbook

Easy, Tasty, and Foolproof Gourmet Recipes to Cook Perfect Meat, Seafood, and Vegetables in Low Temperature for Your Whole Family.

Sophia Marchesi

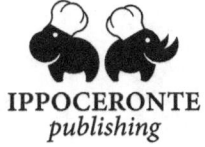

IPPOCERONTE
publishing

Copyright © 2021 by Sophia Marchesi
All rights reserved

This document is geared towards providing exact and reliable information with regards to the topic and issue covered. The publication is sold with the idea that the publisher is not required to render accounting, officially permitted, or otherwise, qualified services. If advice is necessary, legal or professional, a practiced individual in the profession should be ordered.

From a Declaration of Principles which was accepted and approved equally by a Committee of the American Bar Association and a Committee of Publishers and Associations.

In no way is it legal to reproduce, duplicate, or transmit any part of this document in either electronic means or in printed format. Recording of this publication is strictly prohibited and any storage of this document is not allowed unless with the written permission from the publisher. All rights reserved.

The information provided herein is stated to be truthful and consistent, in that liability, in terms of inattention or otherwise, by any usage or abuse of any policies, processes, or directions contained within is the solitary and utter responsibility of the recipient reader. Under no circumstances will any legal responsibility or blame be held against the publisher for any reparation, damages, or monetary loss due to the information herein, either directly or indirectly.

Respective authors own all copyrights not held by the publisher.

The information herein is offered for informational purposes solely and is universal as so. The presentation of the information is without a contract or any type of guarantee assurance.

The trademarks that are used are without any consent, and the publication of the trademark is without permission or backing by the trademark owner. All trademarks and brands within this book are for clarifying purposes only and are owned by the owners themselves, not affiliated with this document.

Cover designed by Rawpixel.com / Freepik, Jade Wulfraat (@jadew) / Unsplash and thiwwy design (@thiwwy)

CONTENTS

INTRODUCTION 7
RECIPES 11
1. Hummus 12
2. Honey Ginger Carrots 14
3. Eggs Benedict 16
4. Ratatouille 18
5. Hokkaido Pumpkin 20
6. Bacon Asparagus 21
7. Baba Ganoush 22
8. Béarnaise Sauce 24
9. Brioche and Eggs 26
10. Overnight Oatmeal with Stewed Fruit Compote 28
11. Cured Salmon 30
12. Pears in Pomegranate Juice 32
13. Garlic Broccoli 34
14. Agnolotti with Artichoke Sauce 36
15. Frittata with Asparagus 38
16. Balsamic Beets 40
17. Cauliflower Alfredo 42
18. Chicken Marsala 44
19. Five Spice Pork 46
20. Smoked Brisket 48
21. Rich and Tasty Duck à Orange 50
22. Lamb Casserole 52
23. Yummy Steak Fries 54
24. Garlic and Rosemary 56
25. Toast with Flawlessly 58
26. Salmon Cakes 60

27. Sweet and Spicy Pork Ribs 62
28. Rich and Creamy Polenta 64
29. Mahi-Mahi Tacos 66
30. Poached Halibut 68
31. Shrimp Cocktail 70
32. Boneless Strip Steak 72
33. Green Soup 74
34. Pumpkin Pie 76
35. Salmon with Hollandaise Sauce 78
36. Lobster Tail with Chimichurri Butter 80
37. Citrus Confit 82
38. Asian Inspired Bok Choy 84
39. Rosemary and Garlic Potatoes 86
40. Turkey and Mushroom Risotto 88
41. Easy Flavor-Packed Pickles 90
42. Carrot and Coriander Soup 92
43. Spicy Korean Pork Ribs 94
44. Apple and Cinnamon Pie 96
45. Dolce De Leche 98
46. Wine and Cinnamon Poached Pears 99
47. Oyster Stew 100
48. Balsamic Mushrooms and Mixed Herbs 102
49. Stracciatella alla Romana Soup 104
50. Caramelized Yogurt with Grilled Berries 106

TEMPERATURE CHARTS 108
COOKING CONVERSION 114
RECIPE INDEX 118

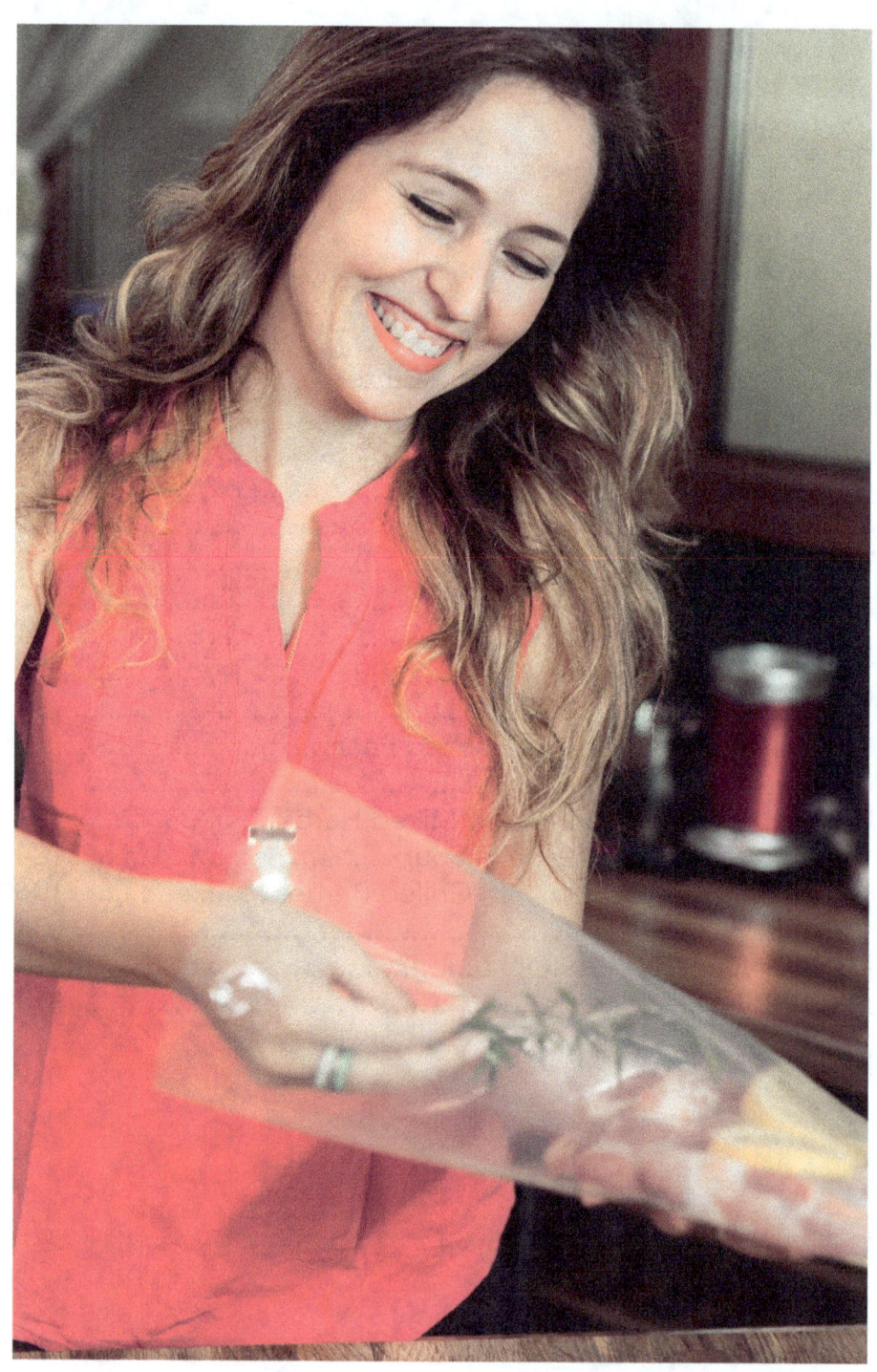

INTRODUCTION

Cooking is something that runs in my blood, most of my food memories are of my Nan cooking Sunday dinners - lasagna and cannelloni to share with the whole family. When I was young, I have never liked to be stuck in a classroom, I started culinary school at a very young age, and the only thing I really wanted was to be out cooking. You could say I was not a particularly good student, but I have always been really passionate about food.

I have been working in a professional kitchen since I was seventeen years old and I'm running my own restaurant since I was 23. The past thirty years have been a rewarding, yet arduous journey that I spent learning the basics and mastering the different cuisines and techniques by taking the best out of each of them. It was last year, during the lockdown, that I realized that I was starting to lose my passion. Preparing a dish had become an aseptic and mechanical where perfection was king.

I wanted to go back to my roots, cooking has always been about my family; preparing a dish together with the people I love gives me time to connect and create precious memories. Setting aside a time where the entire family can work together to create a meal gives us a chance to pause, catch up and just connect with each other.

What I would like to share with you in this book is my renewed passion and a technique that I learned during my time in France, the Sous Vide. This innovative cooking method is something my grandmother never thought existed and creates the perfect opportunity to spend some time in the kitchen with my family. For these reasons, I think the Sous Vide is the perfect combination of my professional and domestic life.

Sous Vide is the French term that translates to "under vacuum" and it is the method for preparing a dish at a specifically controlled temperature and time; your food should be prepared at the temperature at which it will be eaten. Put simply, this procedure involves placing food in vacuum seal bags and boiling it in a specially built bath of water for longer than average cooking times (usually 1 to 7 hours, up to 48 or more in some cases). Cooking at an exact temperature takes the guesswork out of the equation that defines a perfect meal. You can easily prepare your steak, chicken, lamb, pork, etc., exactly the way you like it, every single time.

It is easy to use and leads to great results every time. You will end up with food that is more tender and juicier than anything else you've ever made. This technique will help you to take your everyday cooking to a higher level. To do a top dish, most of the time, you do not need exotic ingredients, it is just a matter to get the best from the ingredients you already know.

The greatest part of Sous Vide cooking is that it does not require your constant presence in the kitchen. When the food is sealed in a bag and placed in the water bath, you can leave it at a low temperature, and it will cook on its own without asking much of your attention. The Sous Vide Cookers that are nowadays available in the market are efficient at regulating the perfect temperature to cook food according to its texture while maintaining the minimum required temperature. So, while your food is in the water, your hands are practically free to work on other important tasks or spend some quality time with your family.

It is an artful skill that is definitely worth trying. If it is just your first time, don't feel bad if you don't get the results you wanted to achieve. You will get better by gaining experience with this cookbook! The key is having patience, the right information, and consistency.

The meals prepared with Sous Vide are tasty and healthy, since this technique does not use added fats during the preparation of your dish also, using low temperature ensures that the perfect cooking point is reached.

Dishes included in this cookbook are simple, delicious, and provide you with so many options that you'll be preparing them for years to come. These recipes are made to be shared with the people you love and to build new precious food memories as I did with my Nan.

RECIPES

1. HUMMUS

Cal.: 244 | Fat: 11g | Protein: 9g

Preparation Time: 11 minutes
Cooking Time: 3 hours
Servings: 6

Ingredients

½ cup dried chickpeas
2 cups water, divided.
2 garlic cloves, divided.
1 tablespoon lemon juice
2 tablespoons tahini
½ teaspoon sea salt
2 tablespoons extra-virgin olive oil
1 teaspoon ground cumin

Directions

1. Fill the water bath with water. Set your machine temperature to 195°F/91°C.

2. Place the chickpeas, 1½ cups water, and 1 garlic clove in a large food-safe zip-top bag. Slowly lower the zip-top bag into the water and, using the water displacement method, the air will escape from the bag. Continue to lower the bag until it is about 1" from being fully Immersed. Once the bag has been

lowered, zip it shut with your fingers.

3. Cook for 3 ½ hours. Check to see if chickpeas are tender and cook longer if needed.

4. Drain the chickpeas and let them cool until they come to room temperature.

5. Using a food processor, pulse the chickpeas, lemon juice, remaining garlic clove, tahini, salt, oil, and cumin. While the food processor is running, slowly pour in the remaining water. Check the texture and thickness of the hummus. If needed, add more water to reach the desired consistency.

6. When ready to serve, scoop the hummus into a small serving bowl and serve with pita bread, crackers, or fresh vegetables.

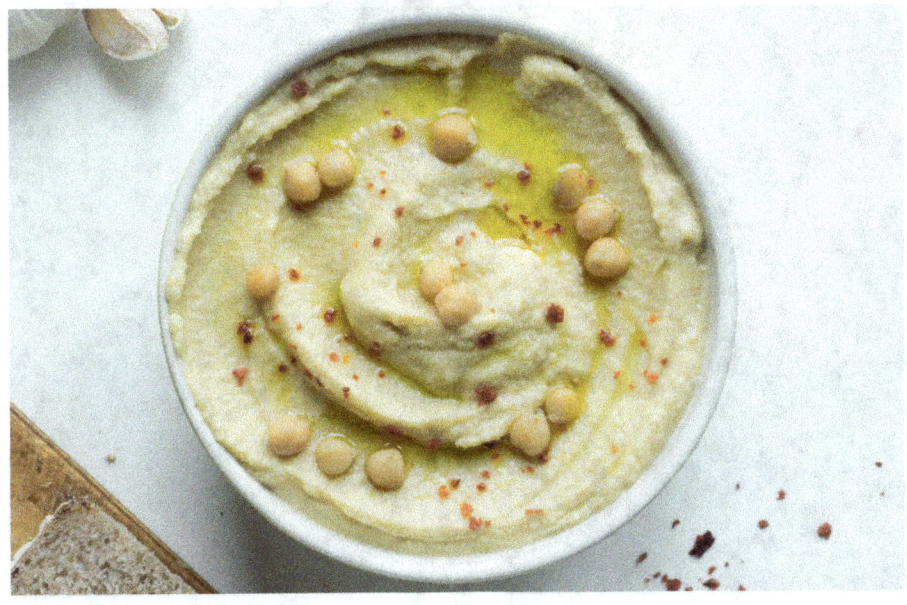

2. HONEY GINGER CARROTS

Cal.: 389 | Fat: 31g | Protein: 22g

Preparation Time: 13 minutes
Cooking Time: 90 minutes
Servings: 4

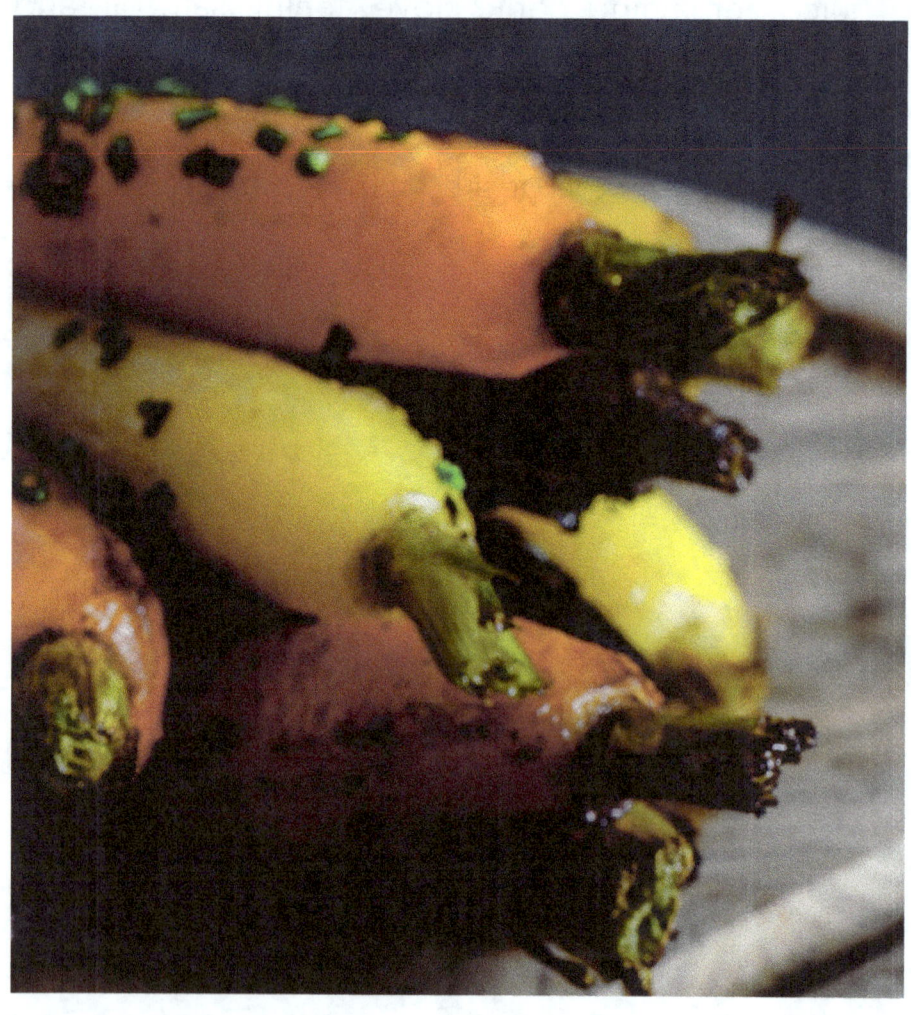

Ingredients

1-pound whole baby carrots, peeled
2 tablespoons butter
2 tablespoons honey
2 teaspoons grated fresh ginger root
1 teaspoon sea salt

Directions

1. Fill the water bath with water. Set your machine temperature to 183°F/84°C.

2. Place the carrots, butter, honey and ginger in a food-safe bag and vacuum seal the bag. Make sure the carrots are lined up side by side and not stacked or piled. Use multiple bags if necessary.

3. Place the carrots in the water bath and cook for 60–90 minutes.

4. Remove the carrots from the bag and place on a serving plate. Sprinkle with sea salt and serve.

3. EGGS BENEDICT

Cal.: 344 | Fat: 21g | Protein: 19g

Preparation Time: 13 minutes
Cooking Time: 1 hour
Servings: 4

Ingredients

4 English muffins, halved, toasted
8 slices Canadian bacon
A handful of fresh parsley, chopped
8 eggs
Butter, as required
For hollandaise sauce:
8 tablespoons butter
2 teaspoons lemon juice
1 shallot, diced
Salt to taste
Cayenne pepper to taste
2 egg yolks
2 teaspoons water

Directions

1. Preheat the Sous Vide machine to 148°F/64°C.

2. Place the eggs in a vacuum-seal pouch or Ziploc bag. Place all the ingredients for hollandaise sauce into another bag. Vacuum seal the pouches.

3. Immerse both pouches in the water bath and set the timer for 1 hour.

4. Meanwhile, cook the bacon in a pan to the desired doneness. Keep warm in an oven along with muffins if desired.

5. Remove the pouches from the water bath. Transfer the contents of the sauce into a blender and blend until smooth.

6. Place muffins on individual serving plates. Crack an egg on each muffin and place on the bottom half of the muffins.

7. Spoon hollandaise over the eggs and garnish with parsley. Cover with the top half of the muffins and serve.

4. RATATOUILLE

Cal.: 411 | Fat: 34g | Protein: 23g

Preparation Time: 11 minutes
Cooking Time: 3 hours
Servings: 4

Ingredients

2 tablespoons olive oil
1 medium sweet onion, diced
1 medium green bell pepper, cored and diced
2 garlic cloves, minced
2 cups peeled and cubed eggplant, no larger than ½" pieces
2 cups cubed zucchini, no larger than ½" pieces
2 medium tomatoes, diced
1 teaspoon sea salt
1 teaspoon dried marjoram or tarragon
½ teaspoon freshly ground black pepper

Directions

1. In a medium skillet, heat oil over medium heat. Add the onion, pepper, and garlic. Cook until the onions are transparent, and the peppers are soft, about 5–7 minutes. Cool to room temperature.

2. Fill the water bath with water. Set your machine temperature to 183°F/84°C.

3. In a large bowl, toss together the sautéed onion and pepper with all the remaining ingredients. Dump the mixture into a food-safe bag and vacuum seal the bag. Make sure the ratatouille is an even thickness within the bag, about 1–1½" thick. Use multiple bags if necessary.

4. Place the bag in the water bath and cook for 3 hours.

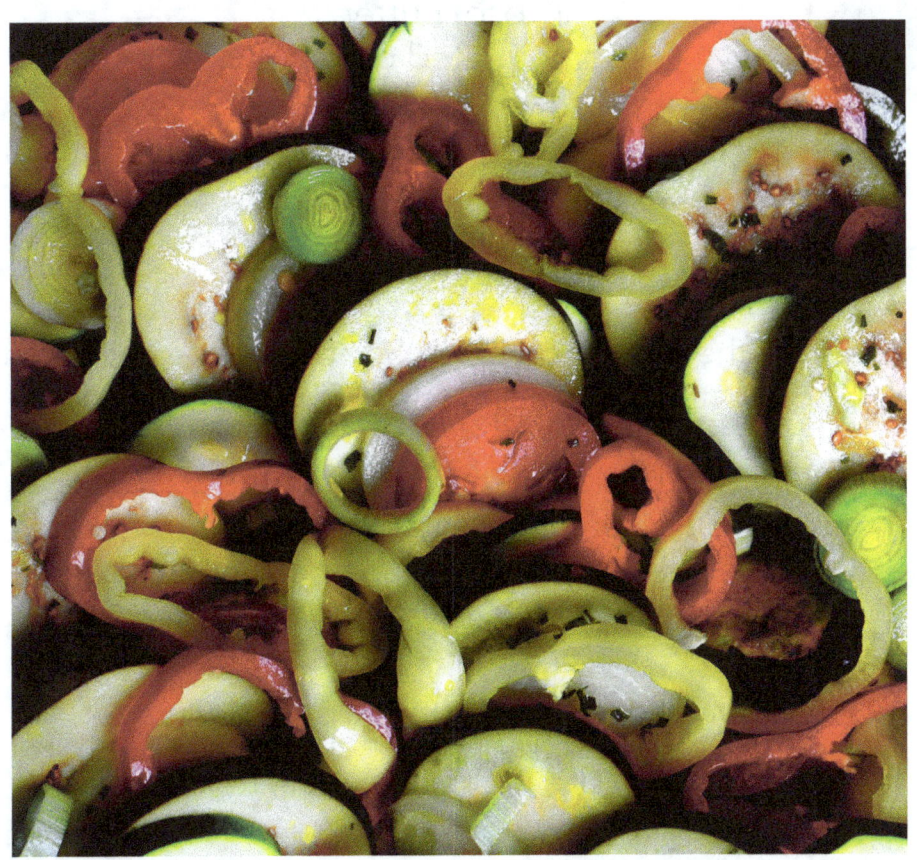

5. HOKKAIDO PUMPKIN

Cal.: 399 | Fat: 31g | Protein: 15g

Preparation Time: 11 minutes
Cooking Time: 20 minutes
Servings: 2

Ingredients

400 g pumpkin meat from Hokkaido
1 tbsp. butter
Some grated ginger
1 tbsp. apple juice
1 pinch of salt and pepper each

Directions

1. Cut up the washed pumpkin. Scrape out the seeds with a spoon (these can still be used for other purposes).

2. Cut the Hokkaido with the peel into bite-sized pieces and vacuum seal in a suitable bag with the apple juice, pepper, salt, 1 teaspoon of butter and ginger.

3. Preheat the water bath to 176°F/80°C and cook the pumpkin for 20 minutes .

4. After removing the pumpkin cubes, fry them briefly in hot butter.

6. BACON ASPARAGUS

Cal.: 190 | Fat: 8.1g | Protein: 8.6g

Preparation Time: 15 minutes
Cooking Time: 45 minutes
Servings: 2

Ingredients

½ lb. asparagus, chopped
Salt, to taste
Black pepper, to taste
2 bacon slices, cooked and chopped
2 tablespoons honey
1 teaspoon lemon juice

Directions

1. Prepare and preheat the water bath at 190°F/88°C.

2. Add asparagus and all the ingredients to a zipper-lock bag.

3. Seal the zipper-lock bag using the water immersion method. Place the sealed bag in the bath and cook for 45 minutes.

4. Once done, transfer the asparagus to a plate. Serve.

7. BABA GANOUSH

Cal.: 194 | Fat: 19g | Protein: 10g

Preparation Time: 9 minutes
Cooking Time: 3 hours
Servings: 6

Ingredients

1 large eggplant peeled and cubed.
1 tablespoon lemon juice
2 garlic cloves
2 tablespoons tahini
1 teaspoon sea salt
2 tablespoons extra-virgin olive oil
2 tablespoons chopped fresh cilantro.

Directions

1. Fill the water bath with water. Set your machine temperature to 185°F/85°C.

2. Place the cubed eggplant in a food-safe bag and vacuum seal the bag. Make sure the eggplant is in only 1–2 layers within the bag. Use multiple bags if necessary.

3. Place the eggplant in the water bath and cook for 2–3 hours.

4. Using a food processor, pulse the cooked eggplant, lemon juice, garlic, tahini, salt and olive oil. Process until smooth and creamy.

5. Add the cilantro and pulse a few times or until it is evenly mixed throughout the dip. Serve.

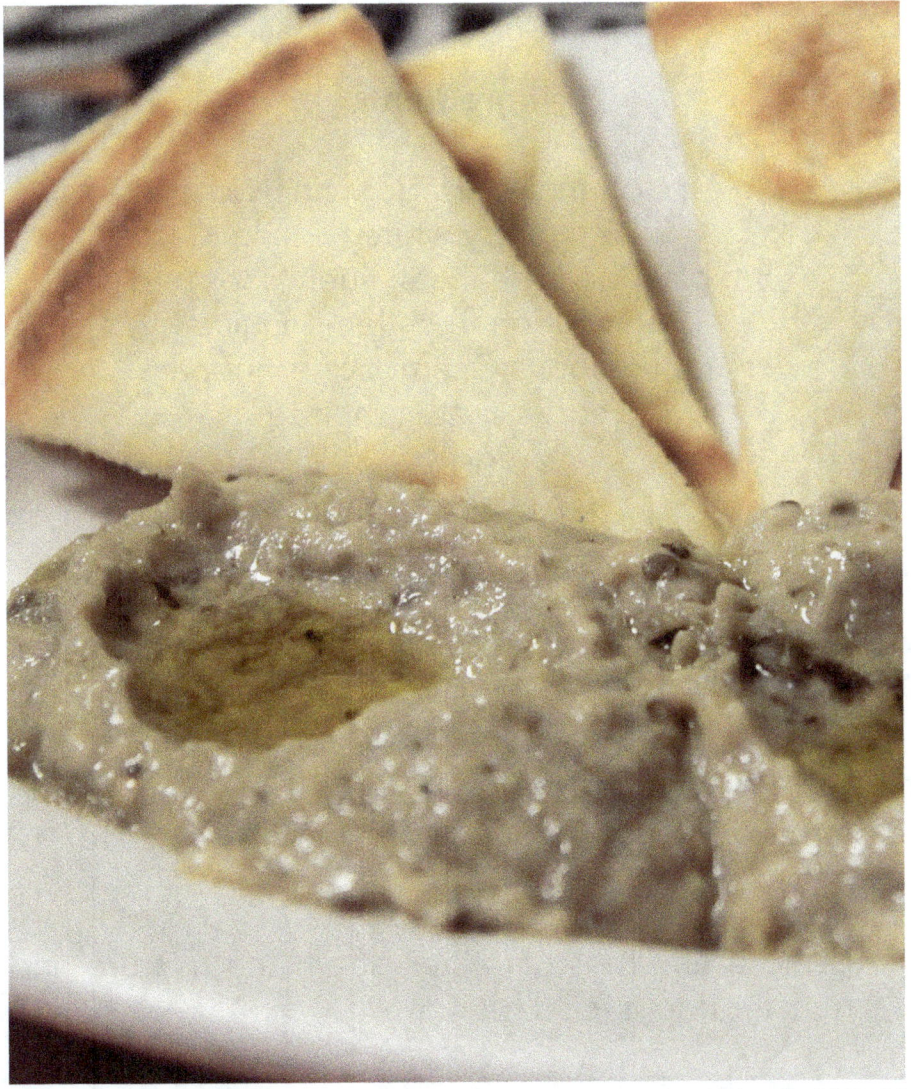

Photo: "Baba ganoush and pita.jpg" by takaokun is licensed under CC BY 2.0

8. BÉARNAISE SAUCE

Cal.: 175 | Fat: 12g | Protein: 4g

Preparation Time: 10 minutes
Cooking Time: 46 minutes
Servings: 12

Ingredients

1 tablespoon fresh tarragon, finely chopped
½ cup dry white wine
3 tablespoons shallots, finely chopped
1 tablespoon fresh lemon juice
4 tablespoons Champagne vinegar
2 sticks butter, melted
5 egg yolks

Directions

1. Prepare your sous-vide water bath to a temperature of 148°F/64°C.

2. Get a pan and add the shallots, wine, vinegar and tarragon. Bring to a boil and then simmer for 12 minutes.

3. Using a fine-mesh strainer, strain the mixture and transfer it to a food blender.

4. Add the egg yolks and blend until completely smooth.

5. Put the sauce into a cooking pouch and immerse it into the preheated water bath.

6. Cook for 25 minutes.

7. Once done, remove the pouch from the water bath and transfer the contents to a bowl.

8. Add the lemon juice and butter and blend until smooth.

9. Serve and enjoy with your choice of roasted vegetable bites.

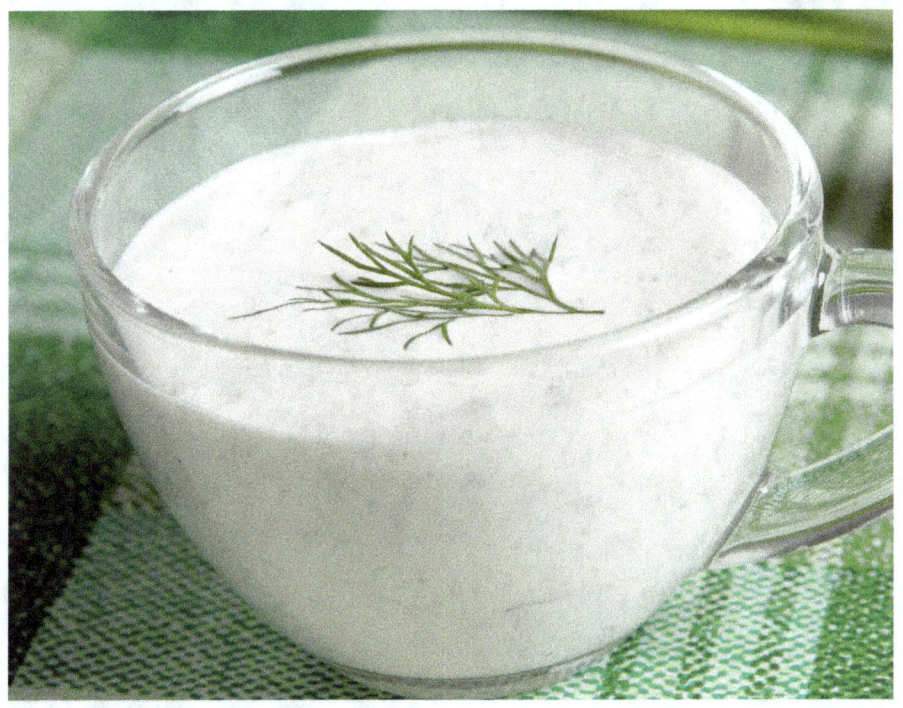

9. BRIOCHE AND EGGS

Cal.: 397 | Fat: 34g | Protein: 19g

Preparation Time: 13 minutes
Cooking Time: 46 minutes
Servings: 6

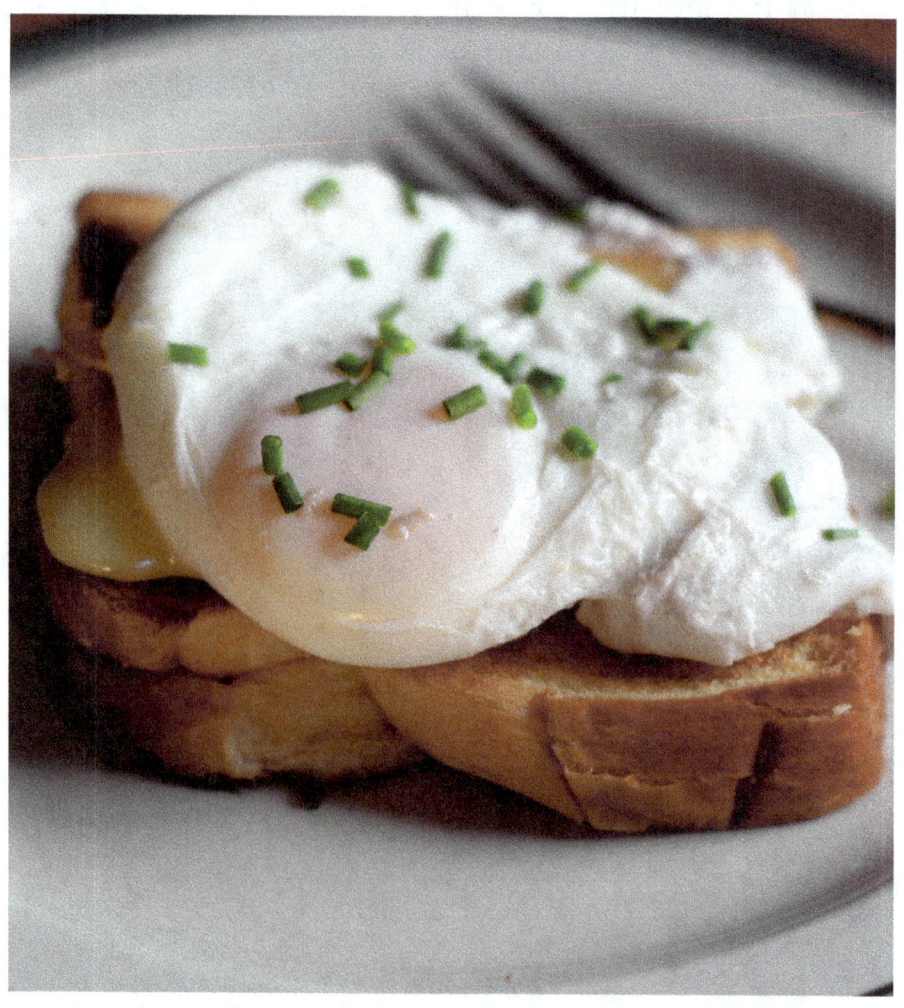

Ingredients

6 brioche buns
6 large eggs
2 scallions, sliced (optional)
1 ½ cups grated cheese

Directions

1. Preheat the Sous Vide machine to 149°F/65°C.

2. Place the eggs on a spoon, one at a time, and gently lower them into the water bath and place on the rack. Set the timer for 45 minutes.

3. When the timer goes off, immediately remove the eggs from the water bath. Place the eggs in a bowl of cold water for a few minutes.

4. Place brioche buns on a baking sheet and break a cooked egg on each bun. Sprinkle cheese on top.

5. Set an oven to broil and place the baking sheet in the oven. Broil for a few minutes until the cheese melts.

10. OVERNIGHT OATMEAL WITH STEWED FRUIT COMPOTE

Cal.: 364 | Fat: 32g | Protein: 19g

Preparation Time: 9 minutes
Cooking Time: 6 hours
Servings: 4

Ingredients

For oatmeal:
2 cups quick-cooking rolled oats
¼ teaspoon ground cinnamon
6 cups water
A pinch salt

For Stewed Fruit Compote:
1½ cups mixed dried fruit of your choice—cherries, apricots, cranberries, etc.
1 cup water
Zest of an orange, finely grated
Zest of a lemon, finely grated
¼ cup white sugar
¼ teaspoon vanilla extract

Directions

1. Preheat the Sous Vide machine to 155°F/68°C.

2. Place oatmeal, water, salt, and cinnamon in a vacuum-seal pouch or Ziploc bag.

3. Place all the ingredients of the fruit compote in another similar pouch and vacuum seal both.

4. Immerse both pouches in the water bath and set the timer for 6 to 10 hours.

5. Remove the pouches and shake them well.

6. Divide the oatmeal into 4 bowls. Top with fruit compote and serve.

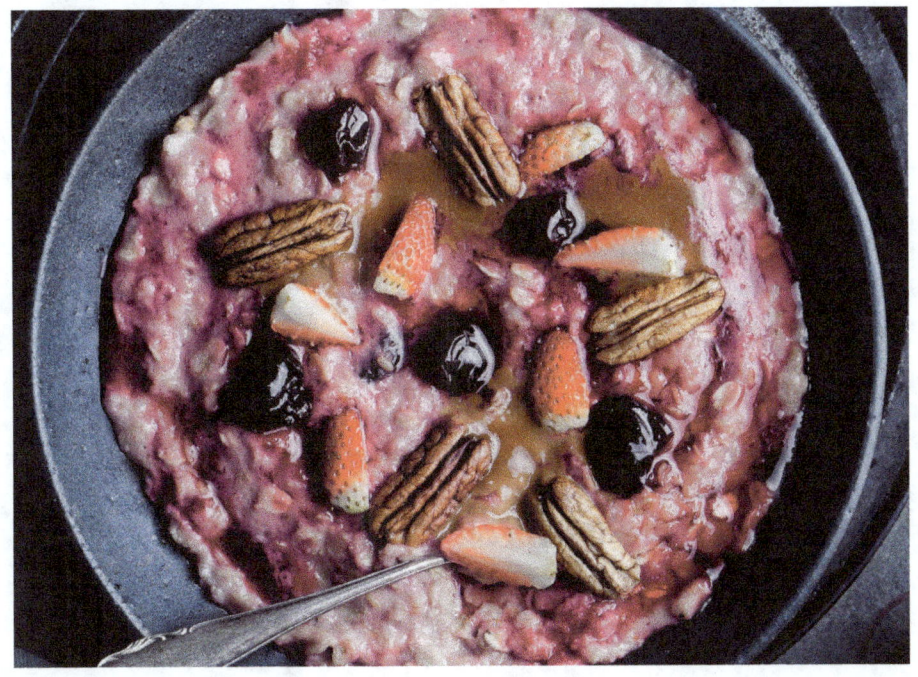

11. CURED SALMON

Cal.: 344 | Fat: 21g | Protein: 19g

Preparation Time: 9 minutes
Cooking Time: 1 hour
Servings: 2

Ingredients

2 salmon fillets (6 ounces each)
8 tablespoons sugar
8 tablespoons salt
2 teaspoons smoke flavor powder (optional)

Directions

1. Take 2 bowls and place a fillet in each bowl.

2. Divide the sugar, salt and smoke flavor powder among the bowls. Mix well. Set aside for 30 minutes.

3. Rinse the fillets in water.

4. Place in a large Ziploc bag. Vacuum seal the pouch.

5. Immerse the pouch in the water bath at 104°F/40°C and adjust the timer for 30 minutes.

6. Just before the timer goes off, make an ice water

bath by filling a large bowl with water and ice.

7. When done, remove the pouch from the water bath and immerse it in the ice water bath. When cooled, remove the pouch from the water bath.

8. Remove the fillets from the pouch and serve.

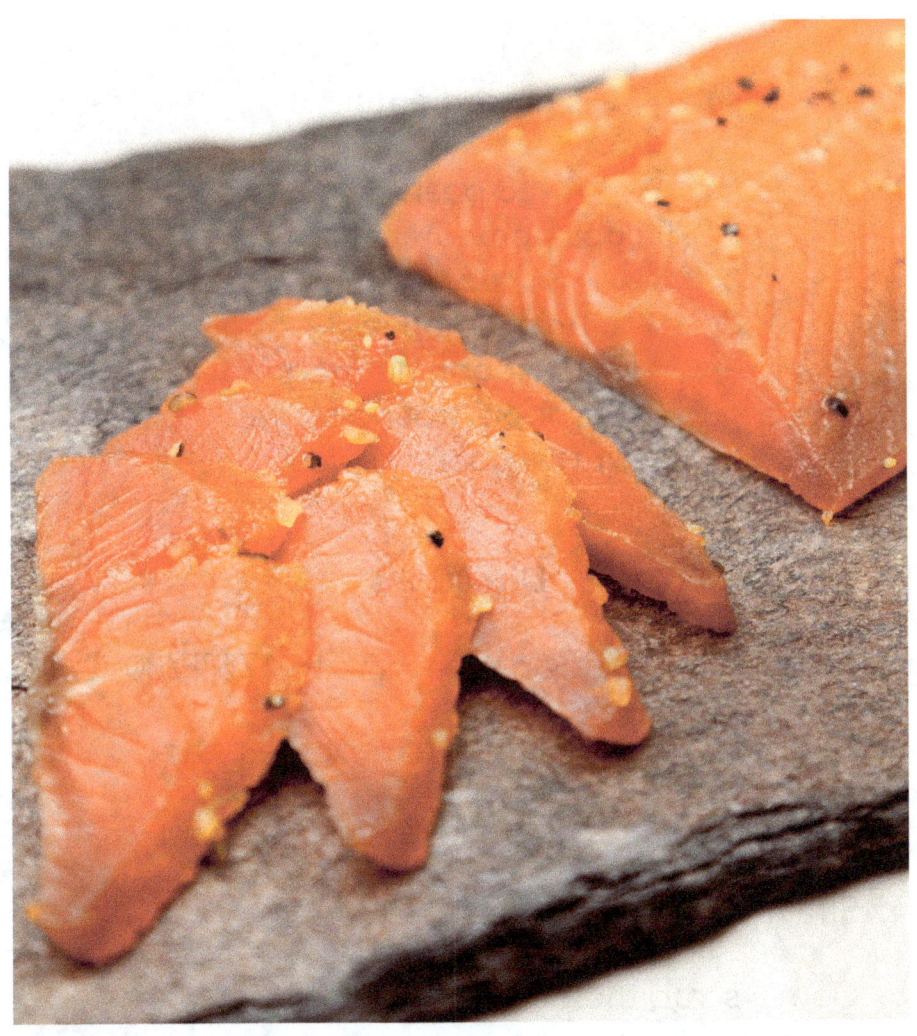

12. PEARS IN POMEGRANATE JUICE

Cal.: 268 | Fat: 0.3g | Protein: 0.8g

Preparation Time: 21 minutes
Cooking Time: 30 minutes
Servings: 8

Ingredients

8 pears
5 cups pomegranate juice
¾ cup sugar
1 cinnamon stick
¼ teaspoon nutmeg
¼ teaspoon ground cloves
¼ teaspoon allspice

Directions

1. Preheat the Sous Vide machine to 176°F/80°C.

2. Combine all ingredients, except the pears.

3. Simmer until the liquid is reduced by half.

4. Strain and place aside.

5. Gently scrub the pears or peel if desired.

6. Place each pear in a bag, and pour in some poaching liquid. Make sure each pear has the same level of poaching liquid.

7. Vacuum seal the pears and Immerse in water.

8. Cook for 30 minutes.

9. Open bags and remove pears carefully. Slice the pears and place onto a plate.

10. Cook the juices in a saucepan until thick.

11. Drizzle over pears and serve warm.

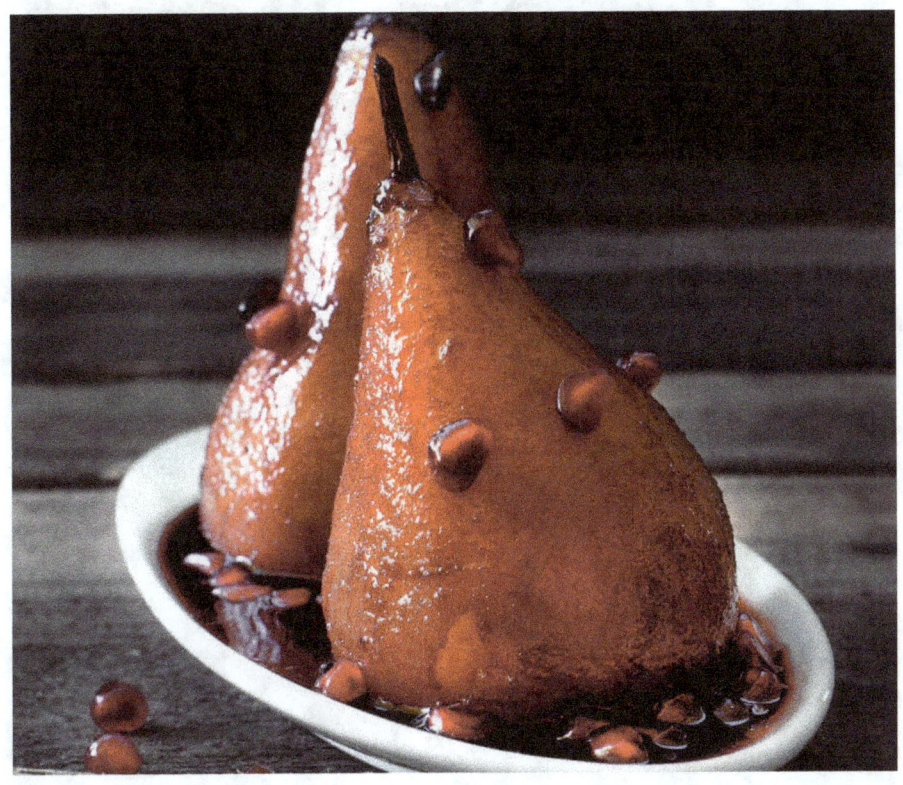

13. GARLIC BROCCOLI

Cal.: 240 | Fat: 25.5g | Protein: 1.6g

Preparation Time: 15 minutes
Cooking Time: 20 minutes
Servings: 2

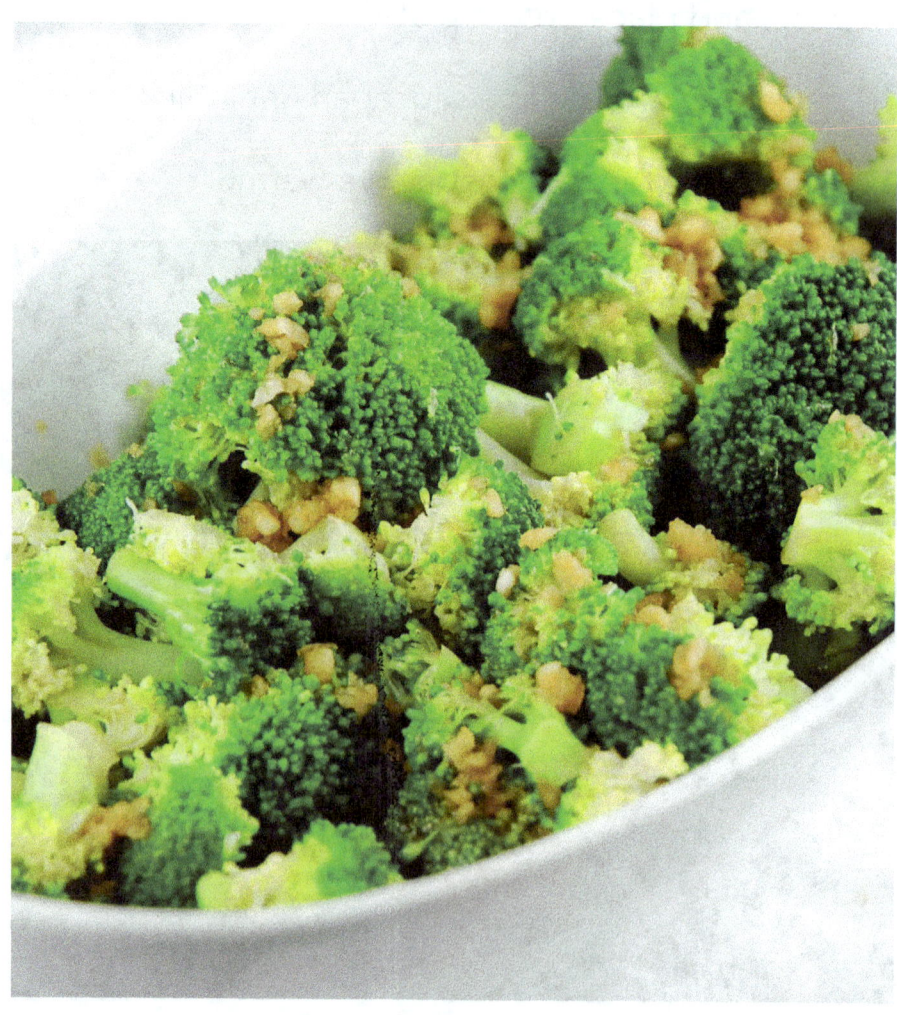

Ingredients

1 broccoli head, cut into florets
3 garlic cloves, peeled
1/4 cup olive oil
1 teaspoon dried rosemary
Salt, to taste
Black pepper, to taste

Directions

1. Prepare and preheat the water bath at 194°F/90°C.

2. Add broccoli and all the ingredients to a zipper-lock bag.

3. Seal the zipper-lock bag using the water immersion method.

4. Place the sealed bag in the bath and cook for 20 minutes.

5. Once done, transfer the broccoli along with the sauce to a plate.

6. Serve.

14. AGNOLOTTI WITH ARTICHOKE SAUCE

Cal.: 525 | Fat: 27.6g | Protein: 475g

Preparation Time: 15 minutes
Cooking Time: 30 minutes
Servings: 4

Ingredients

Sauce:
1 (9-ounce) package frozen artichoke hearts, thawed and coarsely chopped
1 cup frozen peas (do not thaw)
1 cup half-and-half
1 garlic clove, smashed
1/8 teaspoon red pepper flakes
1 teaspoon finely grated lemon zest
2 teaspoons fresh lemon juice
Salt

Pasta:
1 pound refrigerated cheese Agnolotti (or ravioli)
1 cup grated parmesan cheese
1/4 cup fresh basil leaves, chopped

Directions

1. Combine the artichokes, half-and-half, garlic, red pepper flakes and 1/4 teaspoon salt in a vacuum-sealed bag.

2. Set your immersion circulator to 165°F/73.8° and put the bag in the water bath for 30 minutes.

3. While the sauce is cooking, bring a pot of water to a boil and add the agnolotti. Drain the pasta, but retain ½ of the pasta water.

4. Heat a pan over medium heat, and when the sauce is finished in the immersion circulator, remove the bag from the water and pour the contents into the skillet. Add the pasta and ½ cup pasta water and stir to coat. Then add the parmesan cheese and stir. Serve topped with the chopped basil.

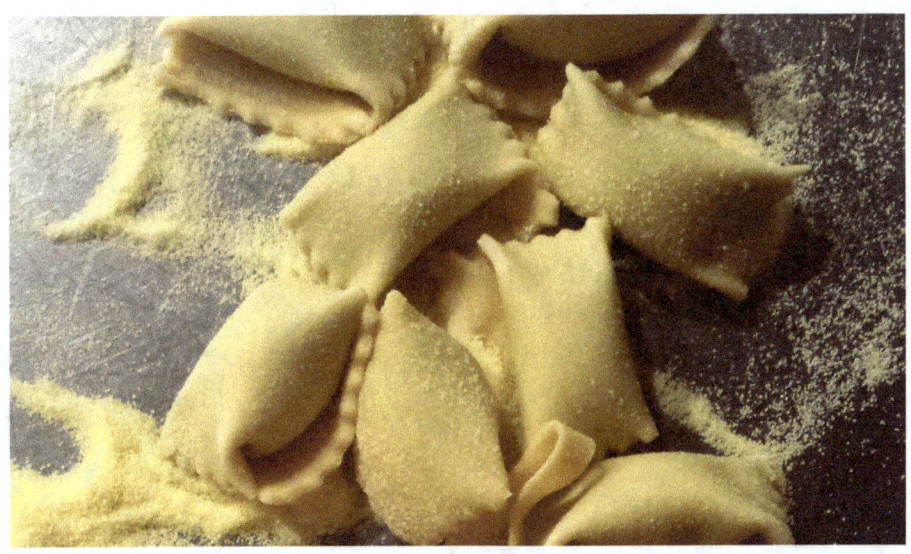

15. FRITTATA WITH ASPARAGUS

Cal.: 383 | Fat: 31g | Protein: 23g

Preparation Time: 10 minutes
Cooking Time: 1 hour
Servings: 3

Ingredients

6 large eggs
2 tablespoons whipping cream
1/4 teaspoon freshly ground black pepper
1 tablespoon olive oil
1 tablespoon butter
12 ounces asparagus, trimmed, cut into 1/4 to ½-inch pieces
1 tomato, seeded, diced
2 teaspoons salt
3 ounces fontina, diced

Directions

1. Heat your immersion circulator to 176°F/80°C.

2. While the water is coming up to temperature, heat a pan over medium heat adding the olive oil.

3. When oil is hot, add the asparagus, salt, pepper and tomato. Sauté until the asparagus is tender and remove from heat.

4. Beat the eggs and pour into a vacuum-sealed bag. Add the contents of the pan along with the butter and diced fontina. Immerse the bag into the water and try to keep it flat on the bottom of the container.

5. Cook for 1 hour, and remove from the water bath. Cut the bag open and serve.

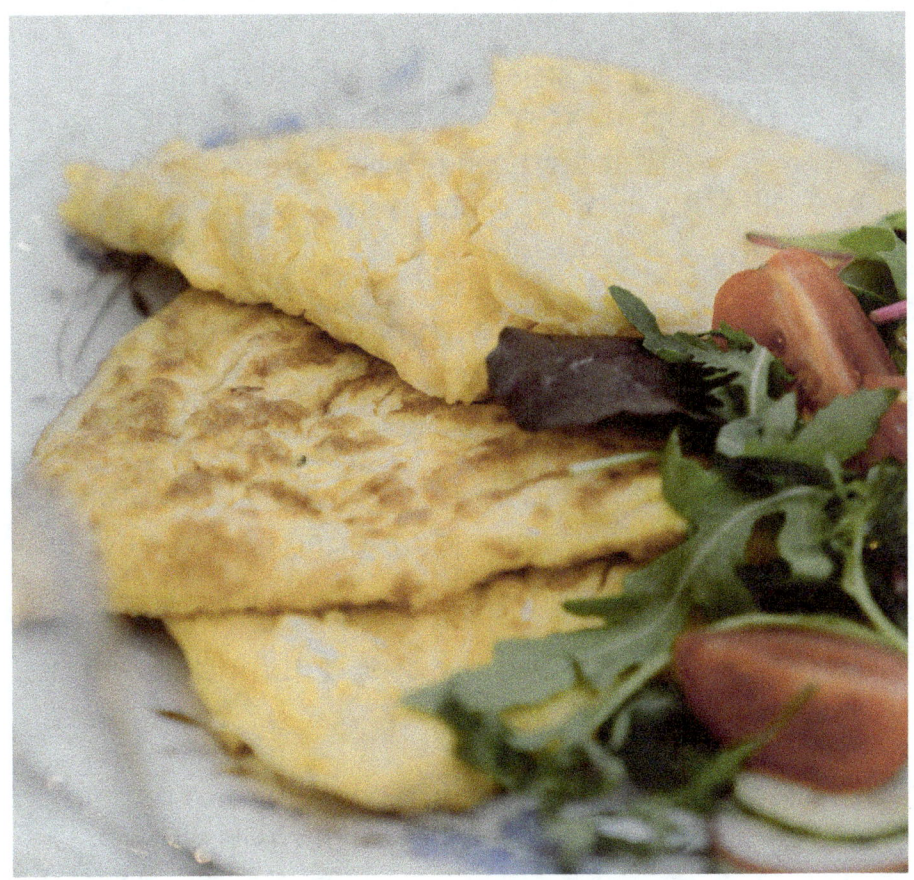

16. BALSAMIC BEETS

Cal.: 74 | Fat: 4.8g | Protein: 0.8g

Preparation Time: 10 minutes
Cooking Time: 2 hours
Servings: 6

Ingredients

6 medium beets (2 bunches, or about 3-½ pounds)
1 teaspoon salt
2 tablespoons extra virgin olive oil
1/3 cup inexpensive balsamic vinegar
1 tablespoon maple syrup
Freshly ground black pepper, to taste

Directions

1. Set your immersion circulator to 185°F/85°

2. Place the chopped beets, olive oil, salt and 2 tablespoons of balsamic vinegar into a vacuum-sealed bag.

3. Immerse the bag in the water bath and cook for 2 hours.

4. While the beets are cooking, combine the remaining balsamic vinegar and maple syrup in a small saucepan.

5. Heat on medium until the mixture has reduced slightly, making sure not to burn the vinegar.

6. Remove the beets from the water bath and transfer to a medium bowl. Pour balsamic reduction over the beets and stir to coat.

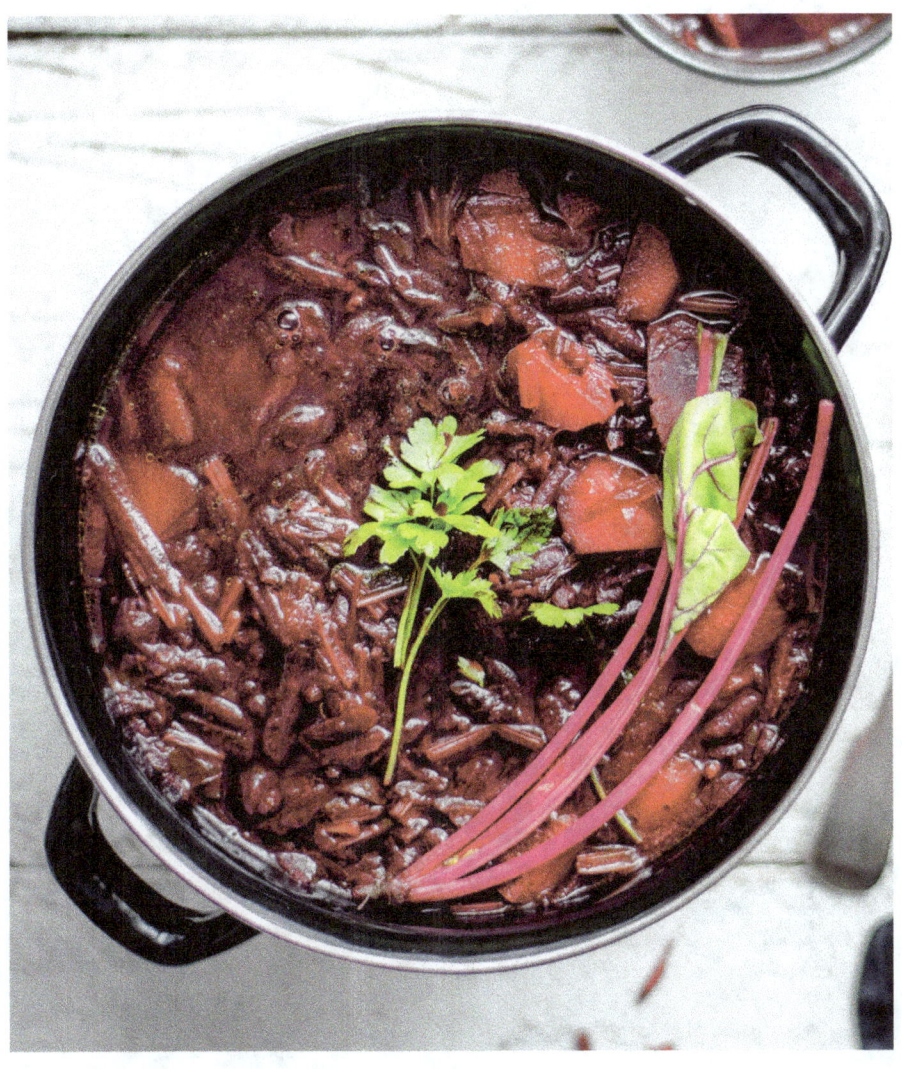

17. CAULIFLOWER ALFREDO

Cal.: 78 | Fat: 5.8g | Protein: 1.3g

Preparation Time: 16 minutes
Cooking Time: 2 hours
Servings: 4

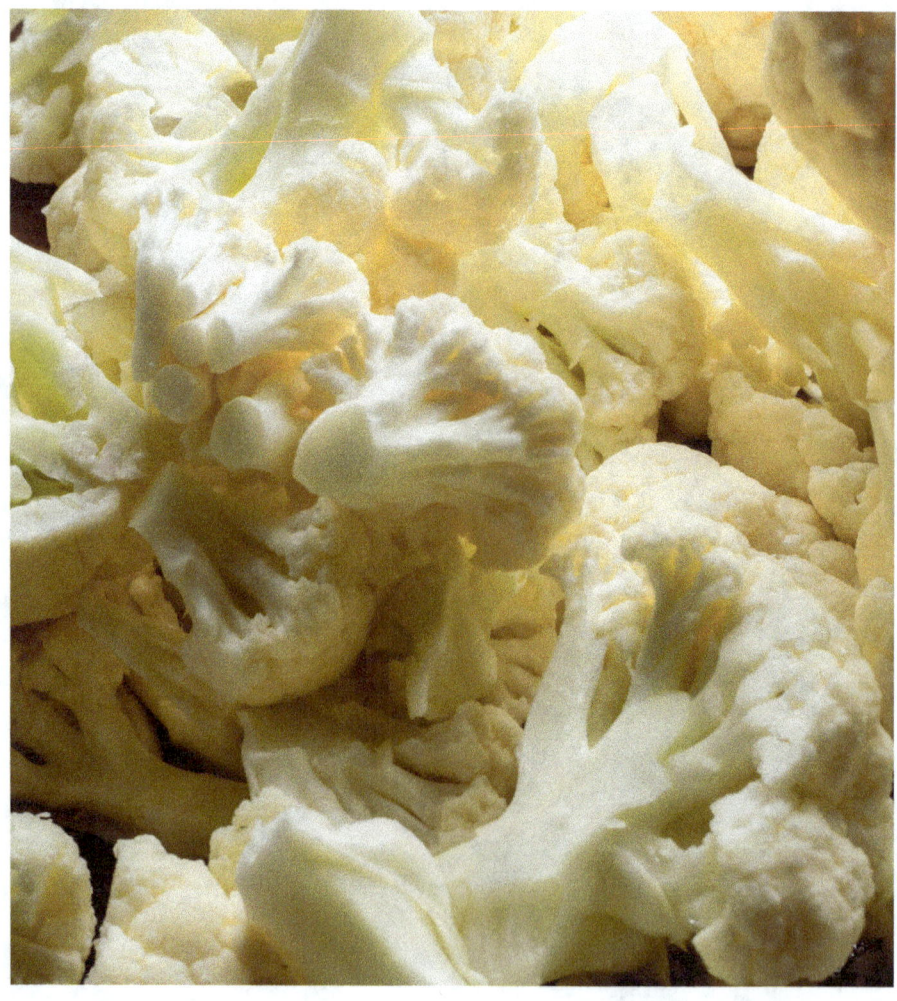

Ingredients

2 cups (400g) chopped cauliflower florets
2 garlic cloves, crushed
2 tablespoons butter
½ cup double-strength chicken stock
2 tablespoons milk
Salt and pepper

Directions

1. Preheat the Sous Vide machine to 185°F/85°C)

2. Place all your ingredients into a Ziploc or vacuum-seal bag. Squeeze out some air and then fold the edge of the bag over to seal.

3. Place the bag into the prepared water bath and clip the edge to the container or pot.

4. Cook for 2 hours.

5. When ready, pour the contents of the bag into a food processor and blend until smooth and creamy.

18. CHICKEN MARSALA

Cal.: 365 | Fat: 1.3g | Protein: 23.2g

Preparation Time: 11 minutes
Cooking Time: 4 hours
Servings: 2

Ingredients

2 boneless, skinless chicken breasts
1 teaspoon salt
1 teaspoon pepper
1 lb. fresh mushrooms, sliced
1 shallot or ½ small onion, diced
2 garlic cloves, minced
1 cup chicken stock
1 cup marsala wine
½ tablespoon flour
1 tablespoon butter
Cooked pasta for serving

Directions

1. Preheat the water bath to 140°F/60°C

2. Salt and pepper the chicken breasts. Place in a bag and add mushrooms. Cook for 2 hours.

3. When chicken is almost cooked, prepare the sauce.

Melt butter in a pan and cook garlic for 30 seconds.

4. Add flour and cook until bubbling subsides, then pour in the stock and wine. Cook until sauce reduces by half. Season to taste.

5. Remove the cooked chicken from the bag then slice and stir chicken and mushrooms into sauce.

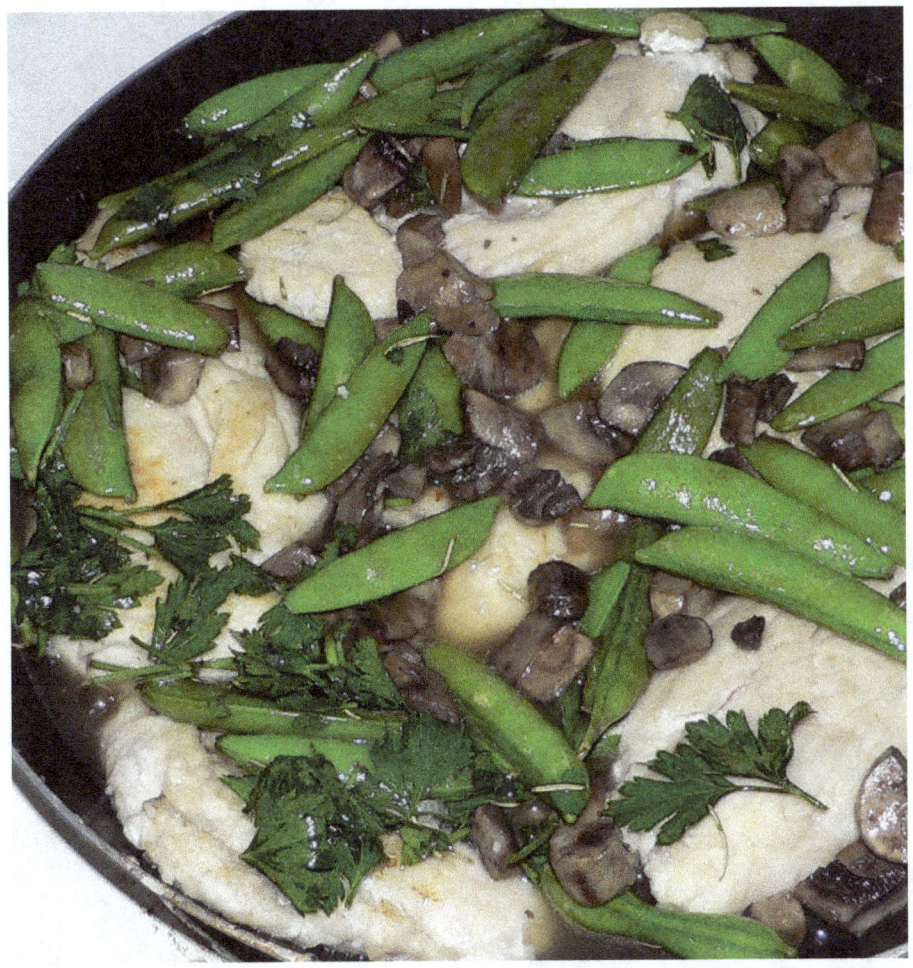

Photo: "Chicken marsala 09.jpg" by Mark Pellegrini (Raul654)

19. FIVE SPICE PORK

Cal.: 549 | Fat: 32g | Protein: 54g

Preparation Time: 5 minutes
Cooking Time: 48 hours
Servings: 4

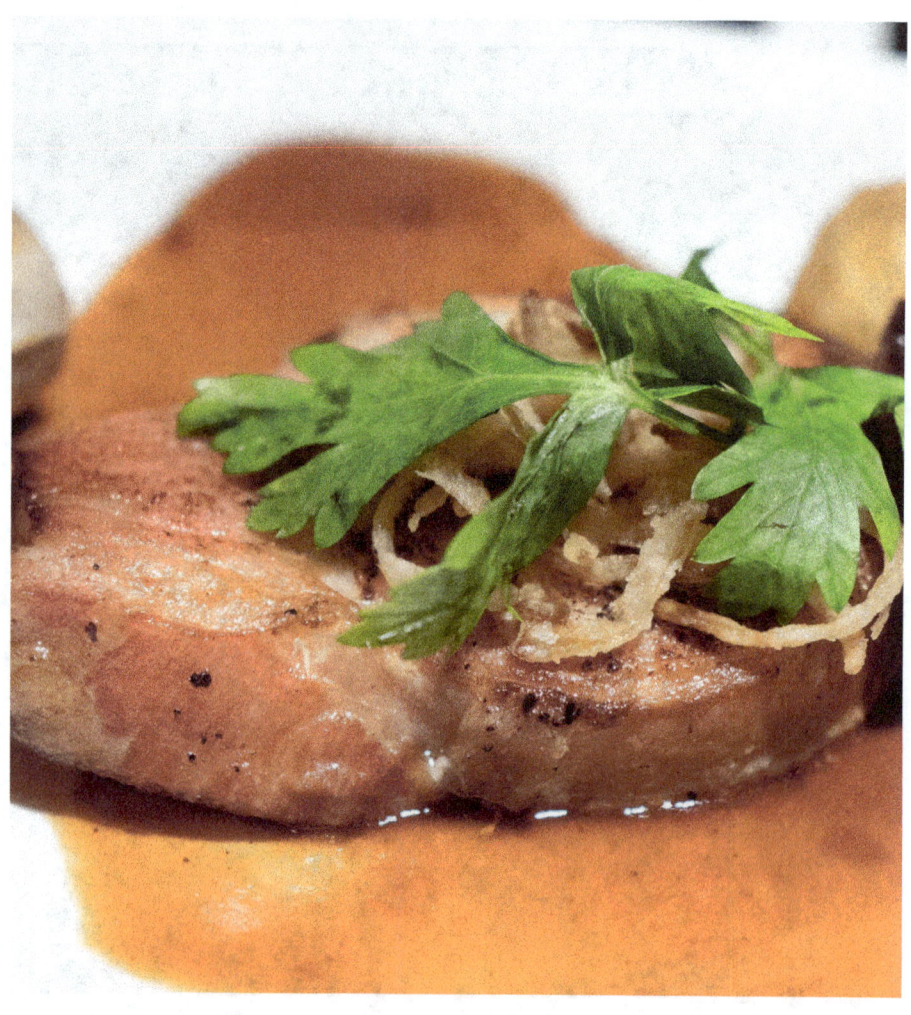

Ingredients

1 lb. pork belly
1 bacon slice
1 tsp. Chinese 5 spice powder
Black pepper
Salt

Directions

1. Preheat the Sous Vide machine to 140°F/60°C.

2. Add pork belly into the Ziploc bag with bacon slice and seasoning.

3. Remove all the air from the bag before sealing.

4. Place the bag into the hot water bath and cook for 48 hours.

5. Remove pork from bag and broil until crisp.

6. Serve and enjoy!

20. SMOKED BRISKET

Cal.: 538 | Fat: 33g | Protein: 50g

Preparation Time: 2 hours 15 minutes
Cooking Time: 38 hours
Servings: 10

Ingredients

2 oz. coarsely ground black peppercorns
2 1/4 oz. kosher salt
1/4 oz. pink salt
1, 5 lb. flat-cut or point-cut brisket
1/4 tsp. liquid smoke

Directions

1. Mix together the different salts and pepper in a bowl. Coat the brisket with about 2/3 of the mixture. Then cut the brisket in half crosswise.

2. Place the 2 briskets in 2 bags, put in 4 drops of liquid smoke in each bag, and seal the bags.

3. Allow the bags to marinate in your refrigerator for 2 to 3 hours

4. Preheat the Sous Vide machine to 155°F/68°C.

5. Place the bag in your preheated water and set the timer

for 36 hours.

6. When the brisket is almost ready, move one of your oven racks to the lower-middle position. Preheat your oven to 300°F/150°C.

7. Use a paper towel to pat the cooked brisket dry. Coat the brisket with the remaining seasoning mixture.

8. Put a wire rack on a baking sheet and place the brisket on top of it with the fat side up. Place the brisket in the oven for about 2 hours. The brisket is done when a dark bark forms on the outside.

9. Place the brisket on a cutting board and use aluminum foil to tent it. Allow the brisket to rest for 30 min. You want the internal temperature to be between 145°F/63°C and 165°F/74°C.

10. Cut the brisket against the grain into desired size pieces and serve.

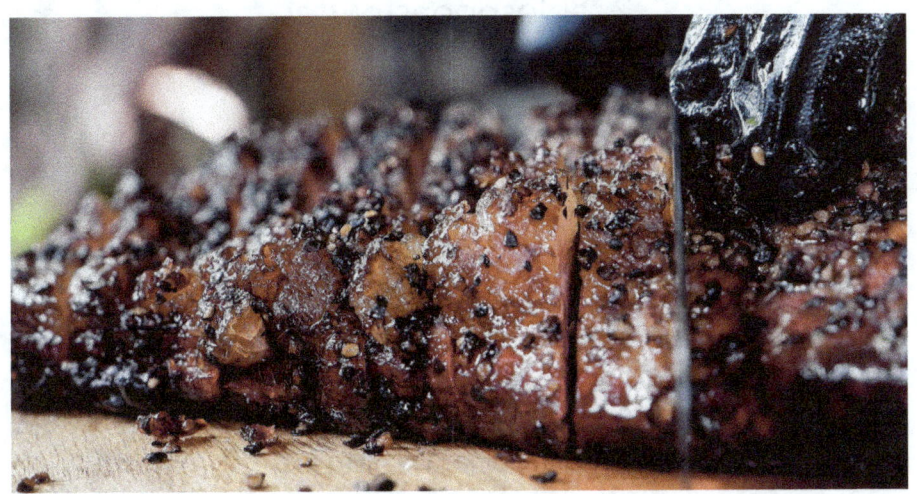

21. RICH AND TASTY DUCK À ORANGE

Cal.: 205 | Fat: 9.3g | Protein: 18.7g

Preparation Time: 21 minutes
Cooking Time: 2 hours 30 minutes
Servings: 4

Ingredients

2 small duck breasts
1 orange, sliced
4 garlic cloves, smashed
1 shallot, smashed
4 thyme sprigs
½ tablespoon black peppercorns
1 tablespoon sherry vinegar
1/4 cup red wine, like Merlot
2 tablespoons butter
Sea salt, to taste

Directions

1. Preheat the water bath to 135°F/57°C.

2. Add the duck breasts with slices of orange, garlic, shallots, thyme and peppercorns to a vacuum bag.

3. Seal and cook for 2 hours 30 minutes.

4. Preheat a frying pan to medium-high heat.

5. Remove duck from the bag and set the bag aside.

6. Fry the duck breast, skin side down, for 30 seconds.

7. Remove the duck breast from the pan and keep warm.

8. Add vinegar and red wine to a frying pan to deglaze leftover fat.

9. Add the contents of the vacuum bag and cook for about 6 minutes over medium heat.

10. Fold in the butter and season with salt and pepper.

11. Slice the duck breast into 2-inch medallions, top with sauce, and serve.

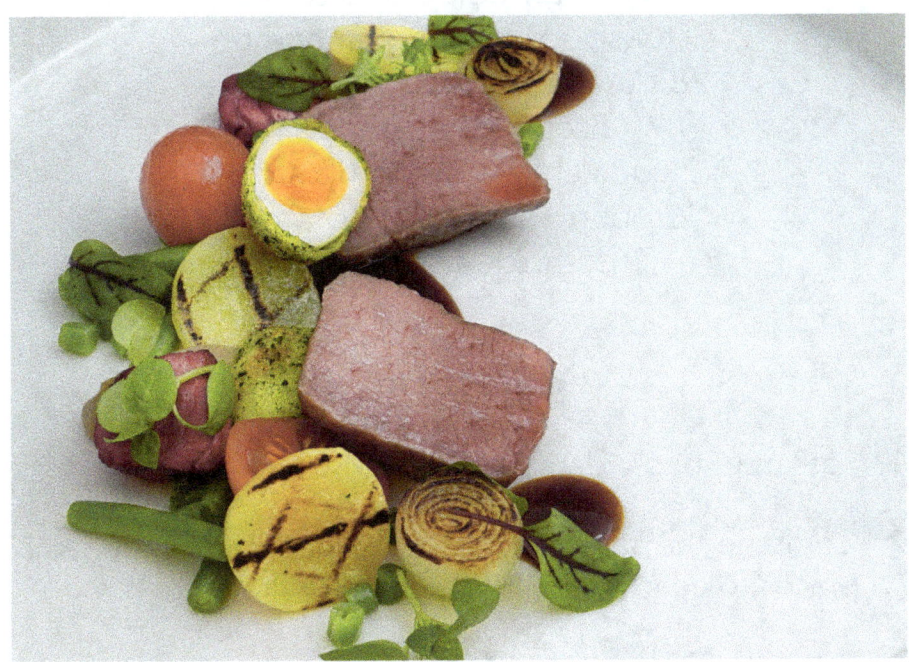

22. LAMB CASSEROLE

Cal.: 434 | Fat: 14.7g | Protein: 50g

Preparation Time: 21 minutes
Cooking Time: 4 hours
Servings: 6

Ingredients

2 tablespoons flour
Salt and pepper
1-½ pounds lamb neck fillet, diced
2 tablespoons vegetable oil
1 medium onion
1 carrot, peeled and diced
1 teaspoon ground cinnamon
28 ounces chopped tomatoes
2 teaspoons honey
2 cups chicken or lamb stock
½ pound small red potatoes
1 package frozen peas

Directions

1. Set your Sous Vide Machine to 180°F/82.2°C.

2. Combine the salt, pepper and flour and toss the lamb pieces to coat. Then, in a medium skillet heat the oil.

3. Brown the lamb on all sides and remove from heat.

4. Add the onion and carrots to the pan and cook for 5 minutes, until lightly browned. Toss in the cinnamon.

5. Transfer the lamb, vegetables and all remaining ingredients to a vacuum-sealed bag.

6. Immerse the bag in the water bath and cook for at least 2 and not more than 4 hours.

7. Remove the bag from the water and pour contents into a casserole dish. The liquid in the bag should have thickened into a nice smooth gravy.

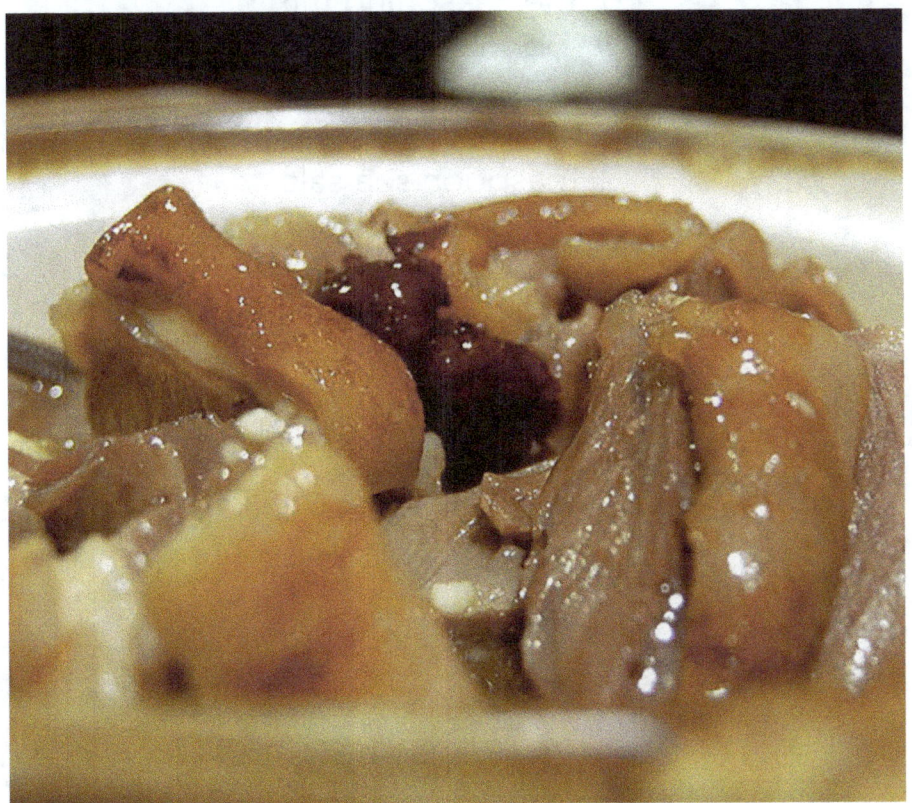

Photo: "Spring lamb casserole" by stu_spivack

23. YUMMY STEAK FRIES

Cal.: 291 | Fat: 11.9g | Protein: 4.9g

Preparation Time: 11 minutes
Cooking Time: 95 minutes
Servings: 4

Ingredients

5 russet Potatoes
½ stick unsalted butter
For the seasoning mix:
1 teaspoon garlic powder
1 teaspoon chili powder
½ teaspoon smoked paprika
½ teaspoon sea salt
½ teaspoon black pepper

Directions

1. Preheat the Sous Vide machine to 190°F/88°C.

2. Cut potatoes in half and lengthwise into wedges.

3. Melt butter in the microwave.

4. Mix together seasonings in a separate bowl.

5. Place potatoes in a resealable plastic bag, toss in butter until covered evenly.

6. Toss in seasoning mix and toss to coat again.

7. Seal and lower bag into the water bath.

8. Cook for 90 minutes.

9. Remove, place on a baking sheet broil for 2-3 minutes on each side.

10. Serve hot!

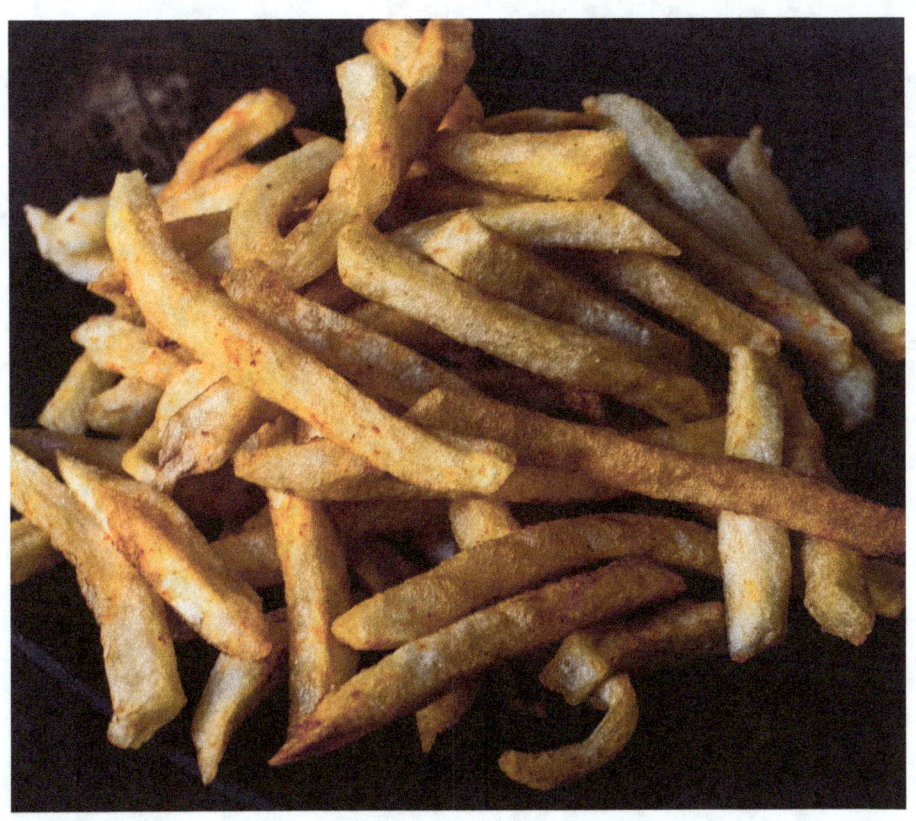

24. GARLIC AND ROSEMARY

Cal.: 228 | Fat: 3.2g | Protein: 7.9g

Preparation Time: 11 minutes
Cooking Time: 46 minutes
Servings: 4

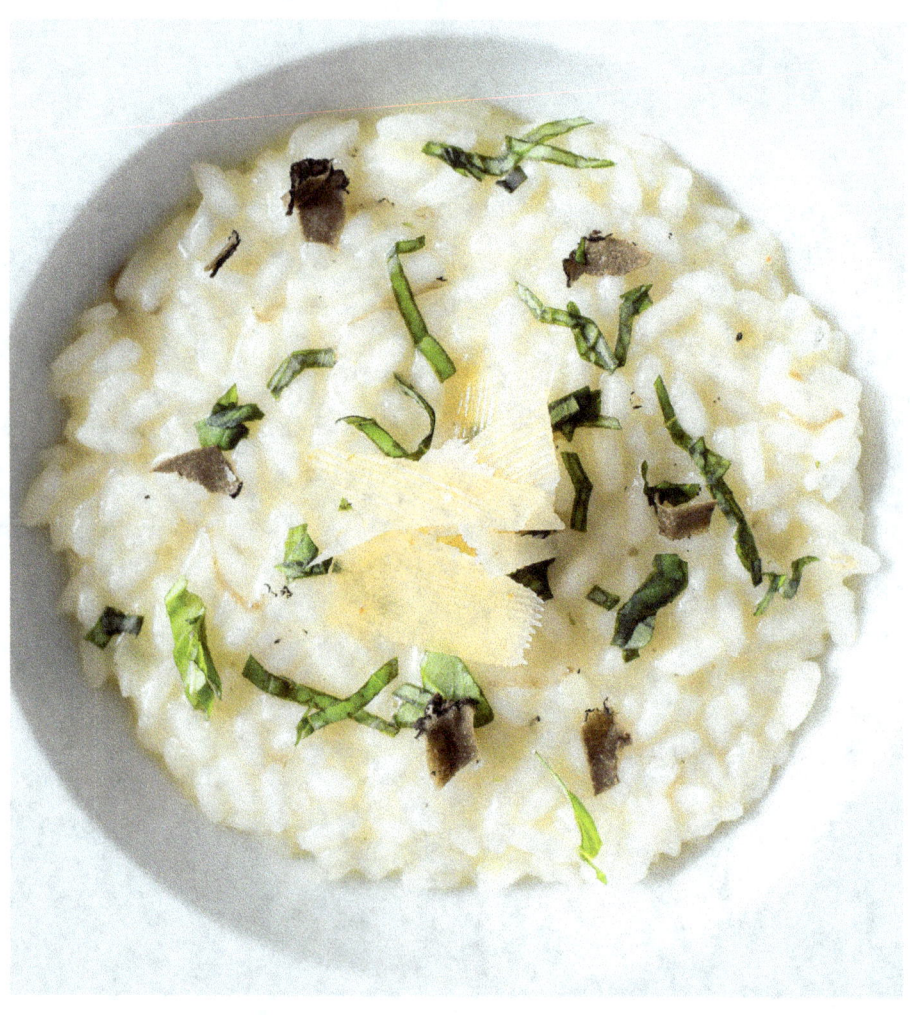

Ingredients

1 cup Arborio rice
1 teaspoon extra virgin olive oil
2 tablespoons jarred, roasted minced garlic
3 cups chicken or vegetable broth
1 sprig of fresh rosemary
Salt and pepper
1/3 cup grated Romano cheese

Directions

1. Preheat the Sous Vide machine to 185°F/85°C. Discard the stems from the rosemary and mince the leaves.

2. Place all ingredients except for cheese in a resealable bag.

3. Place the bag in your preheated container and set your timer for 45 minutes.

4. When the rice is cooked, place it in a bowl and fluff with a fork.

5. Mix in the cheese and serve immediately.

25. TOAST WITH FLAWLESSLY

Cal.: 329 | Fat: 23.41g | Protein: 13.76g

Preparation Time: 11 minutes
Cooking Time: 90 minutes
Servings: 4

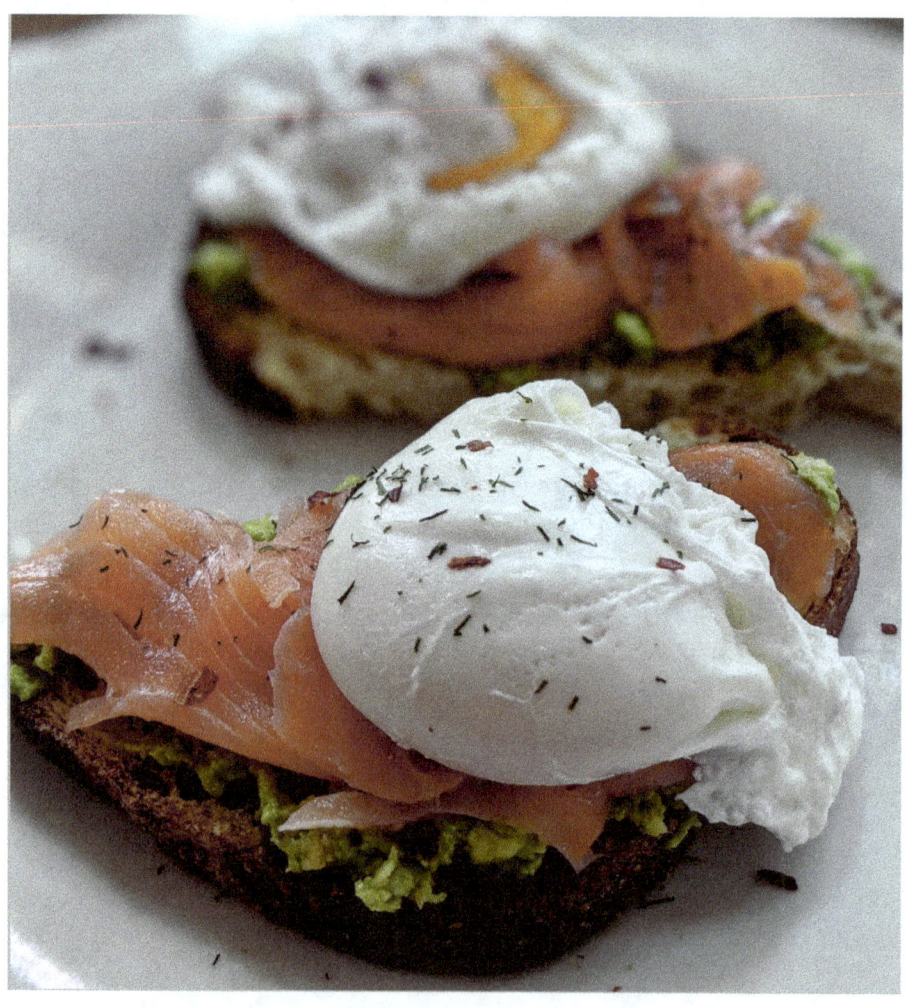

Ingredients

8 large eggs
8 slices of toast
8 slices of smoked salmon/ham
8 slices of tomato
A dash of basil or lettuce leaves, salt and pepper

Directions

1. Preheat a water bath to 64°C/147°F.

2. Put the eggs directly into the bath and cook for 90 minutes.

3. In the meantime, prepare sandwiches, put a smoked salmon or ham on each toast.

4. Top every toast with one slice of tomato and a dash of basil or lettuce leaves.

5. When the eggs are done, remove them from the water bath.

6. Crack each egg on a toast and sprinkle with seasonings.

7. Serve.

26. SALMON CAKES

Cal.: 280 | Fat: 16g | Protein: 17g

Preparation Time: 25 minutes
Cooking Time: 20 minutes
Servings: 6

Ingredients

1 ½ pounds boiled potatoes
1 teaspoon lemon zest
1 teaspoon lemon juice
1 pound chopped salmon
4 tablespoon oil
1 onion
1 tablespoon grated ginger
1 egg
1 teaspoon soy sauce
6 lettuce leaves
Salt, pepper, mayonnaise as per taste

Directions

1. Preheat the Sous Vide machine to 195°F/91°C.

2. Take salmon in the Ziploc bag and remove air.

3. Place this bag in the water bath for 5 minutes.

4. In a pan heat oil and cook the onions and ginger. Add boiled potatoes and mash the mixture.

5. Add salmon, egg, pepper, salt and mix.

6. Make 12 small cakes from this mixture.

7. Heat oil in the skillet and cook these salmon cakes for 6 minutes until brown. Flip and repeat.

8. In a small bowl add lemon juice, soy sauce, ginger, mayonnaise and mix.

9. Serve the salmon cakes with the above mixture.

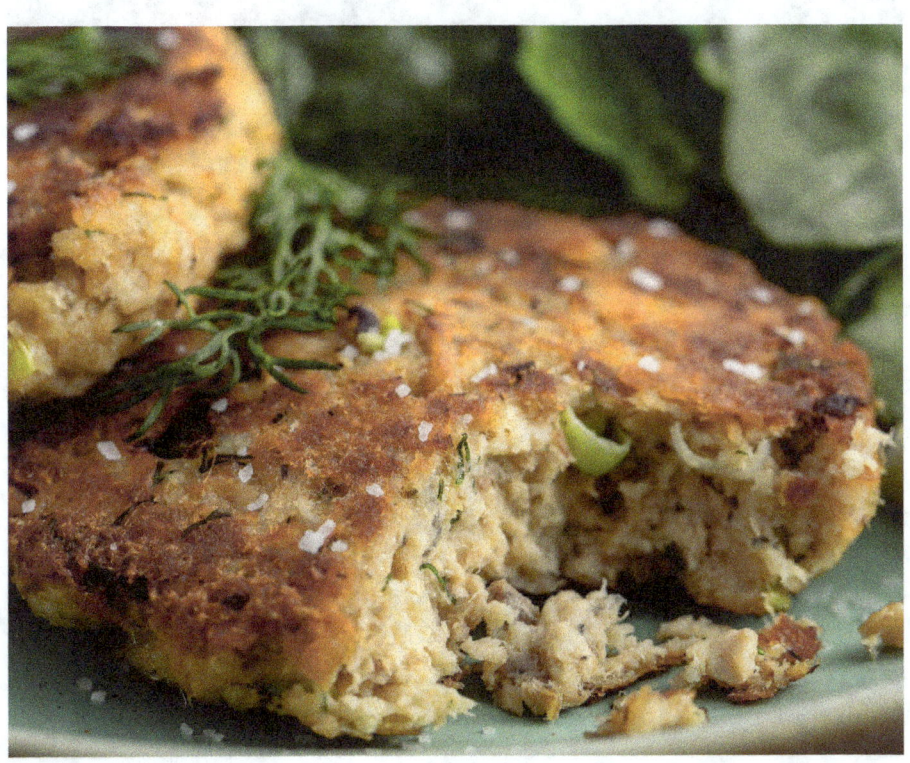

27. SWEET AND SPICY PORK RIBS

Cal.: 880 | Fat: 56g | Protein: 56g

Preparation Time: 11 minutes
Cooking Time: 90 minutes
Servings: 4

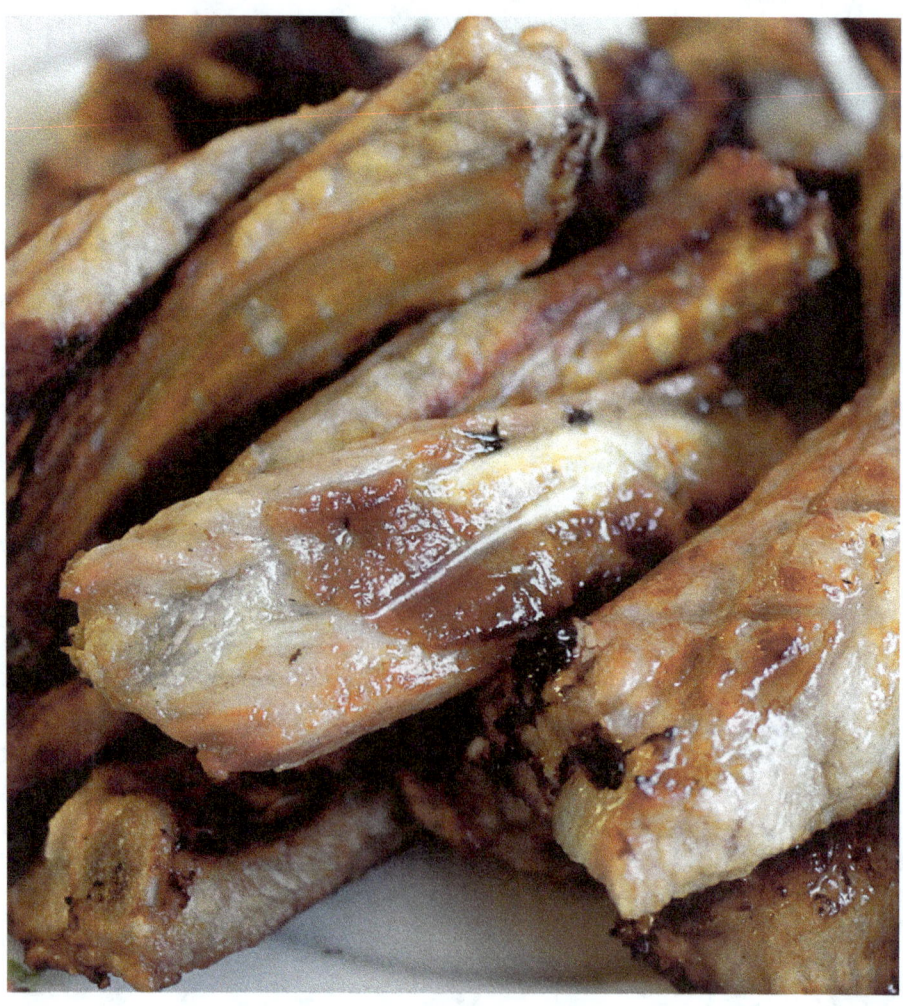

Ingredients

2 full racks baby back pork ribs, cut in half
½ cup jerk seasoning mix

Directions

1. Preheat the Sous Vide machine to 145°F/62°C.

2. Season pork rib rack with half jerk seasoning and place in a large Ziploc bag.

3. Remove all the air from the bag before sealing.

4. Place the bag into the hot water bath and cook for 20 hours.

5. Remove meat from bag and rub with remaining seasoning and place on a baking tray.

6. Broil for 5 minutes. Slice and serve.

28. RICH AND CREAMY POLENTA

Cal.: 176 | Fat: 10.7g | Protein: 15.8g

Preparation Time: 5 minutes
Cooking Time: 1 hour
Servings: 6

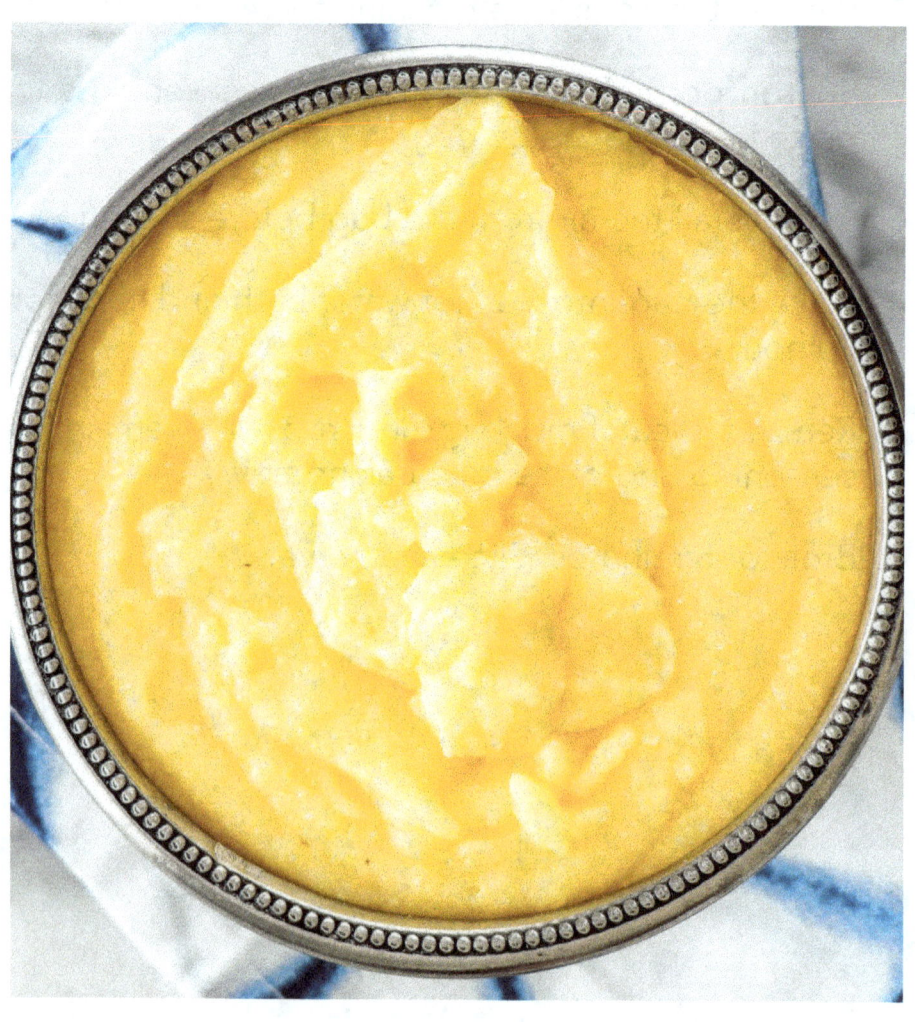

Ingredients

½ cup dry yellow polenta
2 cups chicken or vegetable stock
1/4 cup butter, unsalted
Sea salt
1/4 cup pecorino Romano cheese, for serving

Directions

1. Preheat the water bath to 182°F/83°C.

2. Add polenta, stock, butter and a pinch of sea salt to a resealable plastic bag and seal.

3. Immerse the bag in the water bath and cook for 1 hour.

4. Remove from the water bath and add to a mixing bowl.

5. Fold in cheese until well-incorporated and serve warm.

29. MAHI-MAHI TACOS

Cal.: 300 | Fat: 24g | Protein: 13g

Preparation Time: 15 minutes
Cooking Time: 20 minutes
Servings: 6

Ingredients

1 ½ pound mahi-mahi strips
6 tortillas
1/4 cup cornstarch
1 teaspoon chili powder
½ teaspoon baking powder
1 1/4 cup flour
1 cup beer
Salt, pepper, canola oil

Directions

1. Make a mixture of cornstarch, baking powder, 1 cup flour, salt and chili powder with beer and stand for 10 minutes.

2. Toss the fish strips first in flour and then in the above mixture.

3. Preheat the Sous Vide machine to 195°F/91°C.

4. Take a large Ziploc bag and place these fish strips side by side in it.

5. Apply vacuum to remove the air.

6. Place this bag in the water bath for 20 minutes.

7. Sprinkle salt and pepper and serve on tortillas.

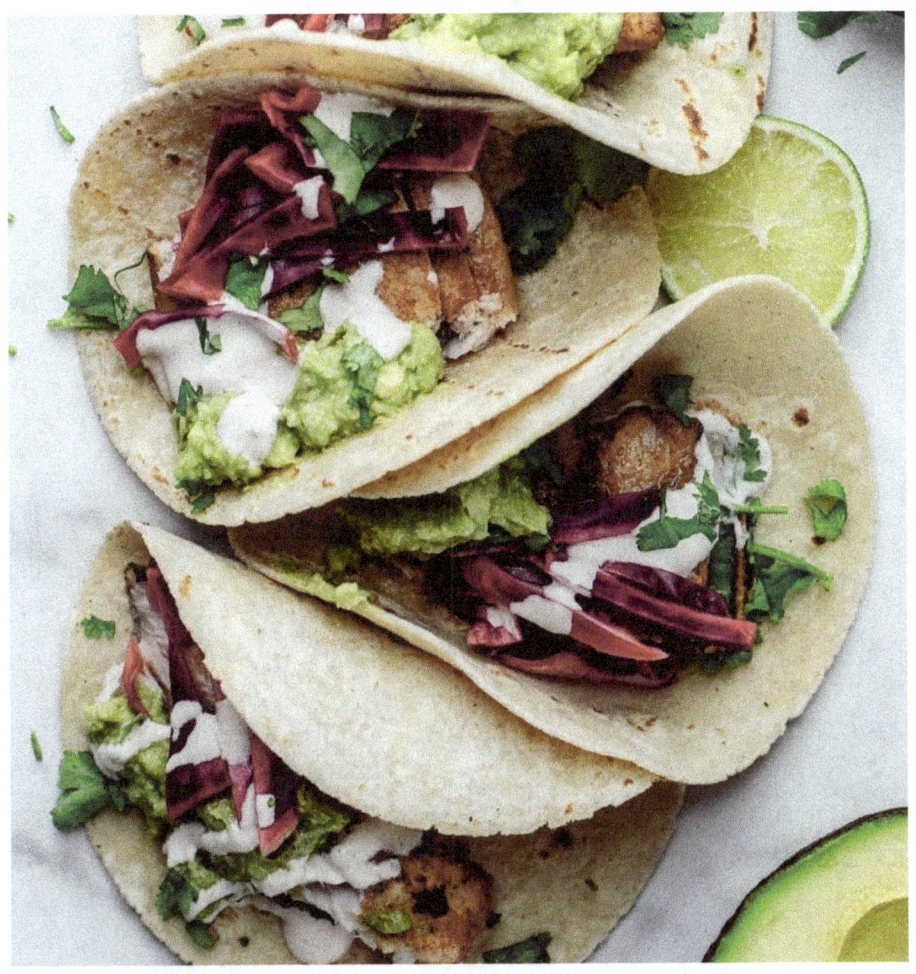

30. POACHED HALIBUT

Cal.: 300 | Fat: 24g | Protein: 13g

Preparation Time: 10 minutes + inactive time
Cooking Time: 30 minutes
Servings: 2

Ingredients

2 5oz. halibut fillets
1/3 cup sea salt
1/3 cup sugar
¼ cup Vin Jaune

Sauce:
½ cup Vin Jaune
¾ cup chicken stock
1 cup unsalted butter
2 tablespoon chopped chives
Salt, to taste

Directions

1. Preheat the Sous Vide machine to 132°F/56°C.

2. Sprinkle the fish fillets with salt and sugar. Place aside minutes.

3. Place the halibut fillets into separate bags. Add Vin Jaune.

4. Vacuum seal the bags and Immerse in water.

5. Cook the fish for 30 minutes.

6. Make the sauce; simmer Vin Jaune and chicken stock in a saucepan until reduced by half.

7. Add the butter and whisk until sauce-like consistency. Season to taste.

8. Remove the fish from the bags and arrange on a plate.

9. Drizzle with sauce and sprinkle with chives.

10. Serve.

31. SHRIMP COCKTAIL

Cal.: 399 | Fat: 31g | Protein: 12g

Preparation Time: 18 minutes
Cooking Time: 30 minutes
Servings: 4

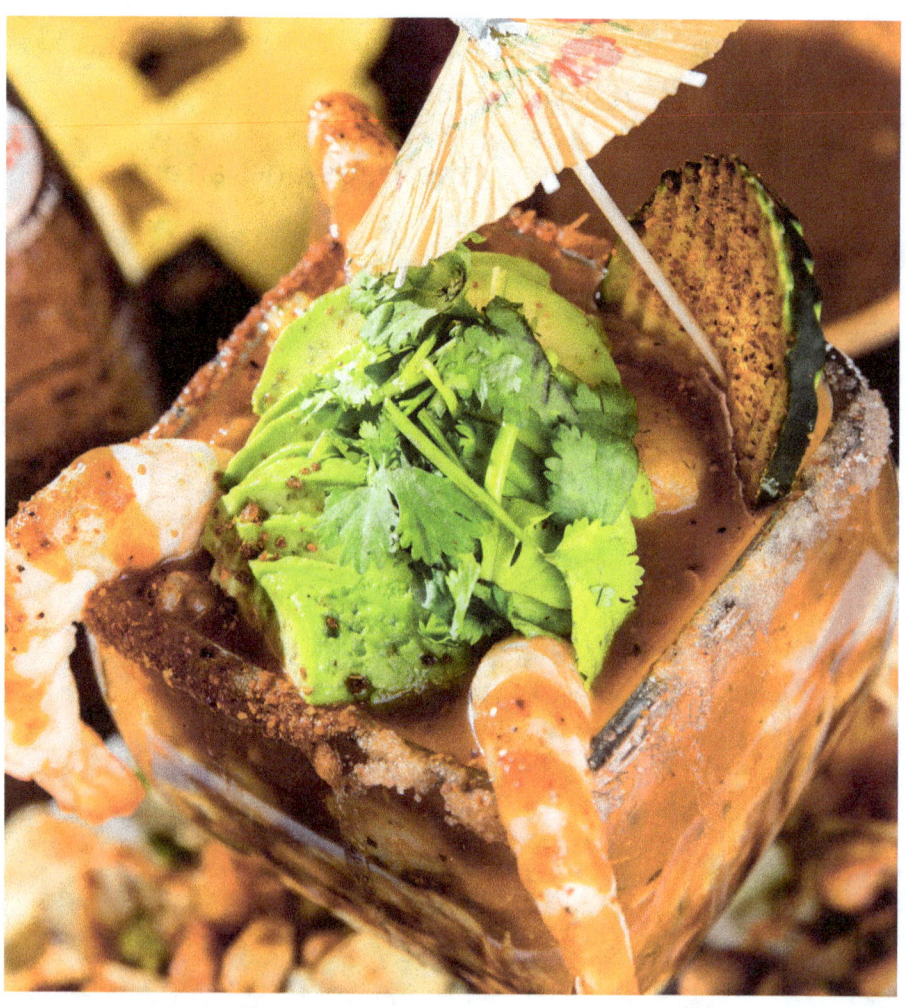

Ingredients

1 pound jumbo shrimp (16-20), peeled and deveined, with tails left on
Cocktail sauce, for serving

Directions

1. Preheat the water bath to 135°F/57°C.

2. Place the shrimp in a large vacuum seal bag. Seal the bag using the vacuum sealer on the moist setting.

3. Place the bag in the water bath and cook for 30 minutes.

4. When finished cooking, remove the bag from the water bath.

5. Transfer bag to an ice bath.

6. When the shrimp are cooled to room temperature, transfer to the refrigerator.

7. Refrigerate for at least 1 hour before serving with the cocktail sauce.

32. BONELESS STRIP STEAK

Cal.: 541 | Fat: 36g | Protein: 57g

Preparation Time: 31 minutes
Cooking Time: 2 hours 30 minutes
Servings: 2

Ingredients

14-16-ounce boneless strip steak, 1½-2 inches thick
¼ tsp. garlic powder
¼ tsp. onion powder
1 tsp. kosher salt, plus more
¼ tsp. freshly ground black pepper, plus more
3 sprigs rosemary
3 sprigs thyme
1 tbsp. grape seed or other neutral oil

Directions

1. Preheat your water bath to 130°F/54.5°C for a medium-rare steak. Change the temperature to 5°F in either direction to adjust wellness.

2. Mix garlic powder, onion powder, 1 tsp. of salt, ¼ tsp. of pepper in a bowl.

3. Rub the mixture all over all 4 sides of the steak. Smack the sprigs of herbs against a cutting board.

4. Place the steak in the bag you're going to use to sous, along with the sprigs of herbs and seal the bag.

5. Place the bag in your preheated water. Set a timer for 2 hours and 30 minutes.

6. When the steak is ready, allow it to rest for 15 minutes.

7. Take the steak out of the bag and let it rest for a few more minutes.

8. While it's resting, season it with salt and pepper to taste.

9. Heat a skittle (ideally cast-iron) on high heat. When it gets really hot, pour in the oil and put in the steak. Let the steak sear for 1 to 2 minutes total, flipping it on all four sides. The steak should form a very nice crust on all sides.

10. Serve immediately.

33. GREEN SOUP

Cal.: 129 | Fat: 5.3g | Protein: 5.8g

Preparation Time: 31 minutes
Cooking Time: 20 minutes
Servings: 6

Ingredients

4 cups vegetable stock
1 tbsp. olive oil
1 garlic clove, crushed
1-inch ginger, sliced
1 tsp. coriander powder
1 large zucchini, diced
3 cups kale
2 cups broccoli, cut into florets
1 lime, juiced and zested

Directions

1. Make a water bath, place it, and set to 185°F/85°C. Place the broccoli, zucchini, kale and parsley in a vacuum-sealable bag. Release air by the water displacement method, seal and Immerse the bag in the water bath. Set the timer for 30 minutes.

2. Once the timer has stopped, remove and unseal the bag. Add the steamed ingredients to a blender

with garlic and ginger. Purée to smooth. Pour the green purée into a pot and add the remaining listed ingredients. Put the pot over medium heat and simmer for 10 minutes.

3. Serve as a light dish.

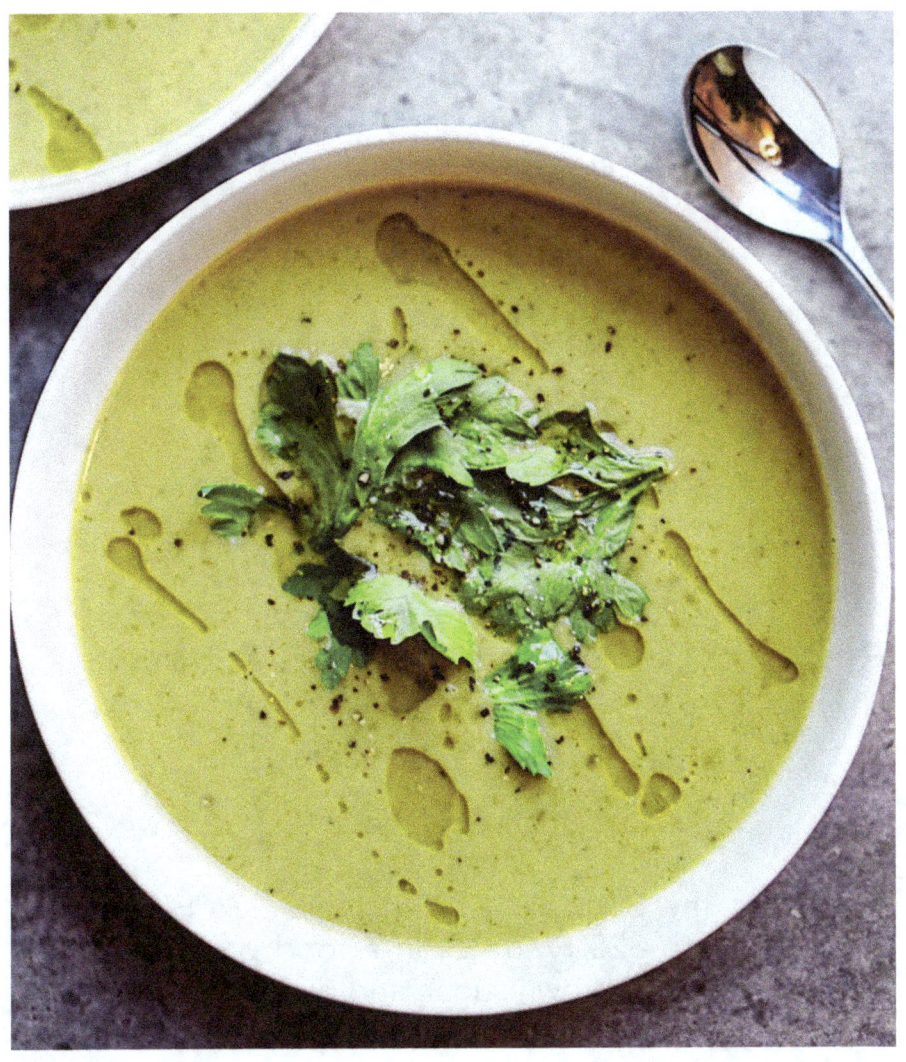

34. PUMPKIN PIE

Cal.: 183 | Fat: 9g | Protein: 22g

Preparation Time: 11 minutes
Cooking Time: 2 hours 8 minutes
Servings: 8

Ingredients

1 cup dark brown sugar
2 cups of canned pumpkin
2/3 cups of heavy cream plus extra for serving
4 large eggs
2 tsp. ground ginger
2/3 cup whole milk
1 tsp. ground nutmeg
2 tsp. ground cinnamon
¼ tsp. ground cloves
½ tsp. salt
2 tbsp. granulated sugar
9 honey graham crackers, broken to medium pieces
5 tbsp. unsalted butter, melted and warm

Directions

1. Preheat the Sous Vide machine to 176°F/80°C and the oven to 325°F/162°C. In a food processor, combine the eggs, brown sugar, and pumpkin. Blend for 1 minute or until the mixture becomes smooth. Transfer

the mixture into a large bowl with a spout. Clean the blade and bowl of the food processor. Add the cloves, salt, nutmeg, cinnamon, ginger, milk, and cream into the bowl with the pumpkin mixture. Stir well until completely combined.

2. Pour the mixture into a zip-lock freezer bag and seal using the water immersion method. Place the freezer bag into the water bath. Cook in the cooker for 90 minutes. Meanwhile, start making the crust by combining sugar and graham crackers in the food processor. Ground the graham crackers for 1 minute or until it turns into fine crumbs.

3. Turn on the food processor and slowly pour the melted butter through the feed tube. Process for 20 seconds or until the texture becomes that of wet sand. Place the graham cracker mixture onto a 9-inch pie plate. Spread the mixture to evenly cover the bottom and sides of the pie plate. Using the bottom of a clean drinking glass, press the mixture to make a compact layer. Place the pie plate in the oven and bake for 15-18 minutes or until the crust is golden brown. Once done, place the pie plate on a wire rack to cool completely.

4. Once the cooker timer goes off, remove the freezer bag from the water bath. Place the bag on a plate and let cool at room temperature for 15 minutes. Once cool, cut one corner and pipe the mixture into the cooled pie crust. Smooth the top using a spatula.

5. Place the pie in the refrigerator and chill for at least 8 hours. To serve, let the pie cool down to room temperature before slicing. Serve with freshly whipped cream.

35. SALMON WITH HOLLANDAISE SAUCE

Cal.: 419 | Fat: 37g | Protein: 17g

Preparation Time: 14 minutes
Cooking Time: 76 minutes
Servings: 2

Ingredients

For Salmon:
2 fresh salmon filets
Salt for brining

For Hollandaise:
4 Tbsp. butter
1 Egg yolk
1 tsp. Lemon Juice
1 tsp. Water
½ Shallot, diced
Pinch of cayenne
Salt, to taste

Directions

1. Dry brine salmon by generously salting both sides and place in the refrigerator for a minimum of 30 minutes.

2. Preheat the water bath to 148°F/64°C.

3. Add all of the ingredients for Hollandaise sauce into a large Ziploc bag and seal it using the water displacement method. It will be blended later, so no need to mix it.

4. Immerse and cook for 45 minutes.

5. Decrease your water bath temperature to 130°F/55°C. Note: Add ice or a few cups of cold water to speed this up.

6. Place salmon in a Ziploc bag and seal it using the water displacement method.

7. Cook salmon for 30-45 minutes.

8. Remove your Hollandaise mixture from the water bath and pour it into your blender.

9. Blend on a medium speed until the mixture is a smooth light yellow.

10. Remove salmon, pat dry, and sear (if desired).

11. Serve with hollandaise sauce.

36. LOBSTER TAIL WITH CHIMICHURRI BUTTER

Cal.: 415 | Fat: 25g | Protein: 43.7g

Preparation Time: 11 minutes
Cooking Time: 36 minutes
Servings: 2

Ingredients

4 tbsp. softened unsalted butter
2 tbsp. parsley
2 tsp. fresh lemon juice
1 small garlic clove, finely minced
2 lobster tails, about 8 oz. each
1 lemon, halved
Parsley for garnish

Directions

1. Preheat the Sous Vide machine to 135°F/57°C. Chop the parsley, mince the garlic, and cut the lemon in half.

2. Mix the parsley, lemon juice, garlic and butter in a bowl until well combined.

3. Place the lobster in the bag with half of the butter and cook for 30 minutes.

4. When the lobster is almost finished cooking, preheat your grill so half the grill is on high heat and the other half is medium-low.

5. When the lobster is cooked put them under cold water until cool and cut them in half lengthwise.

6. Place the tails on the hot side of the grill with the flesh side down for 2 minutes. Flip the tails and baste with remaining butter, cooking another 2-3 minutes. Remove the tails from the grill. Allow the lemon pieces to cook on the hot side of the grill with the flesh side down for 2-3 minutes.

7. Garnish the tails with parsley and serve with the grilled lemon.

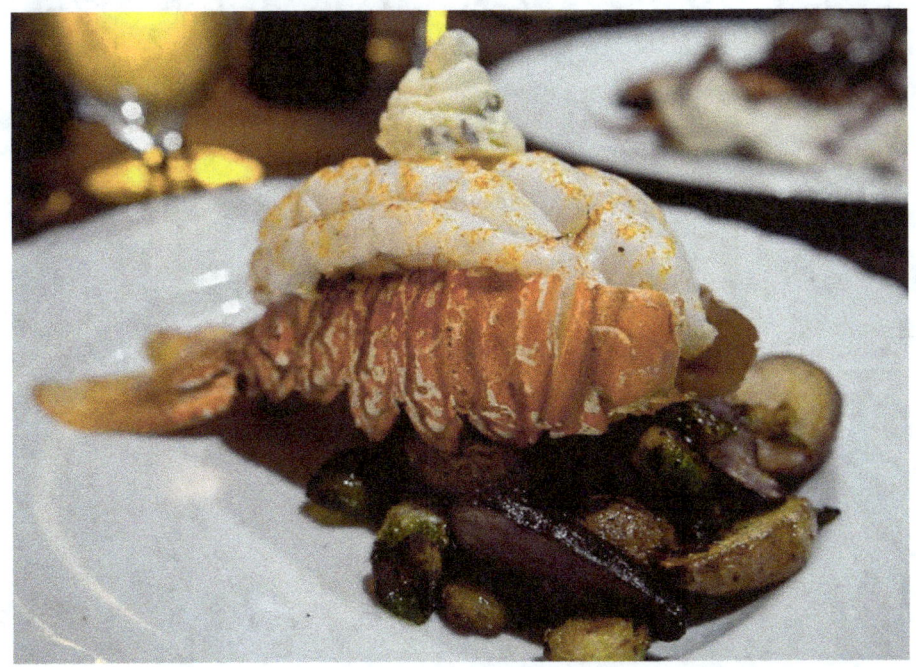

Photo: "New Year's Eve 2011 - Lobster Tail" by Edsel L

37. CITRUS CONFIT

Cal.: 90 | Fat: 1g | Protein: 2g

Preparation Time: 11 minutes
Cooking Time: 60 minutes
Servings: 15

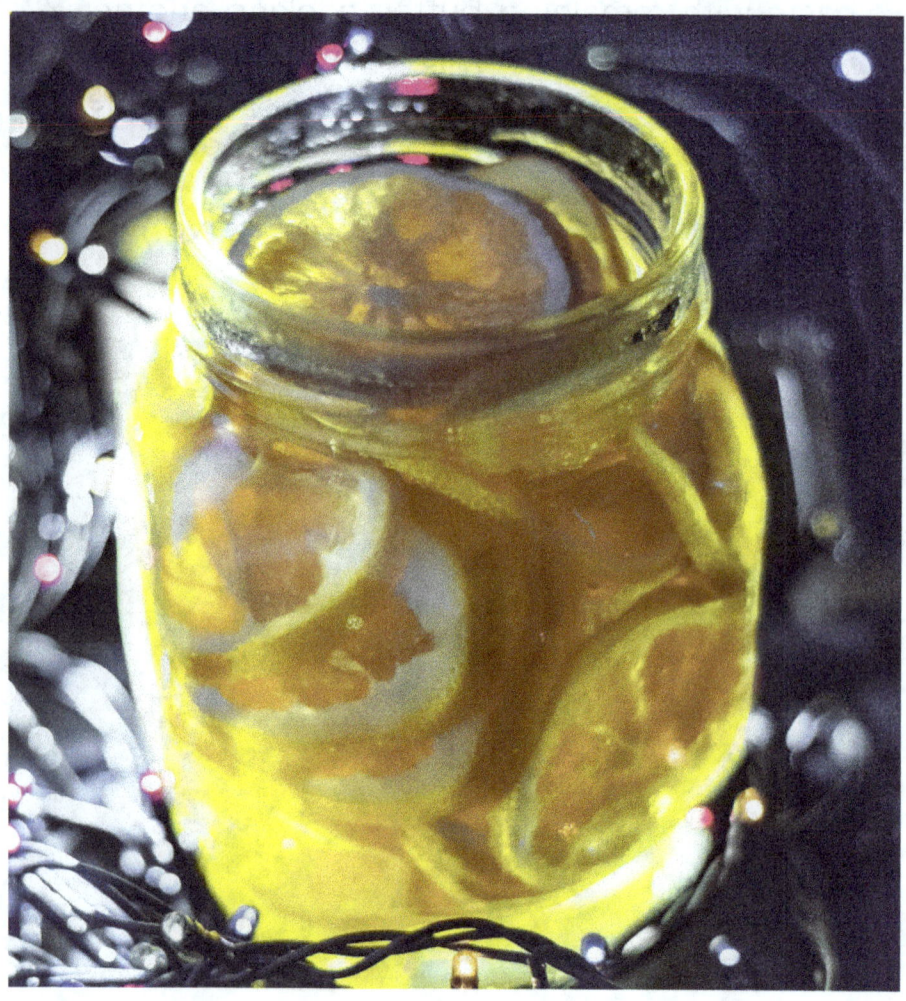

Ingredients

2 lemons, sliced and cut into quarters
1 orange, sliced and cut into quarters
1 lime, sliced and cut into quarters
½ cup sugar
½ cup salt

Directions

1. Preheat the Sous Vide machine to 185°F/85°C.

2. In a big bowl, combine all ingredients and mix well, making sure that fruits are evenly covered with salt and sugar.

3. Carefully put the mixture into the vacuum bag and seal it.

4. Cook for 1 hour in the water bath.

5. This confit is very rich in vitamins and can be stored in the fridge for at least 1 month.

38. ASIAN INSPIRED BOK CHOY

Cal.: 98 | Fat: 1g | Protein: 9g

Preparation Time: 11 minutes
Cooking Time: 30 minutes
Servings: 4

Ingredients

1 tbsp. ginger, minced
2 garlic cloves, minced
1 tbsp. toasted sesame oil
1 tbsp. canola oil
1 tbsp. soy sauce
1 tbsp. fish sauce
1 tsp. red pepper flake
1 lb. baby bok choy, cut in half lengthwise
1 tbsp. toasted sesame seed
1 tbsp. cilantro leaves

Directions

1. Preheat the Sous Vide machine to 176°F/80°C.

2. Put the garlic and ginger in a large heat-proof container.

3. Put the sesame oil and canola oil in a small pot and heat it on medium heat. You want the oil to get so

hot that it just starts to smoke.

4. Take the pot off the heat and pour it into the container with the garlic and ginger.

5. Mix in the bok choy, red pepper flakes, fish sauce and soy sauce.

6. Place the entire mixture in the bag you're going to use to sous and seal the bag.

7. Place the bag in your preheated water and set the timer for 20 minutes.

8. Place the cooked bok choy on a plate or in a bowl, and top with the cilantro and sesame seeds.

9. Serve immediately.

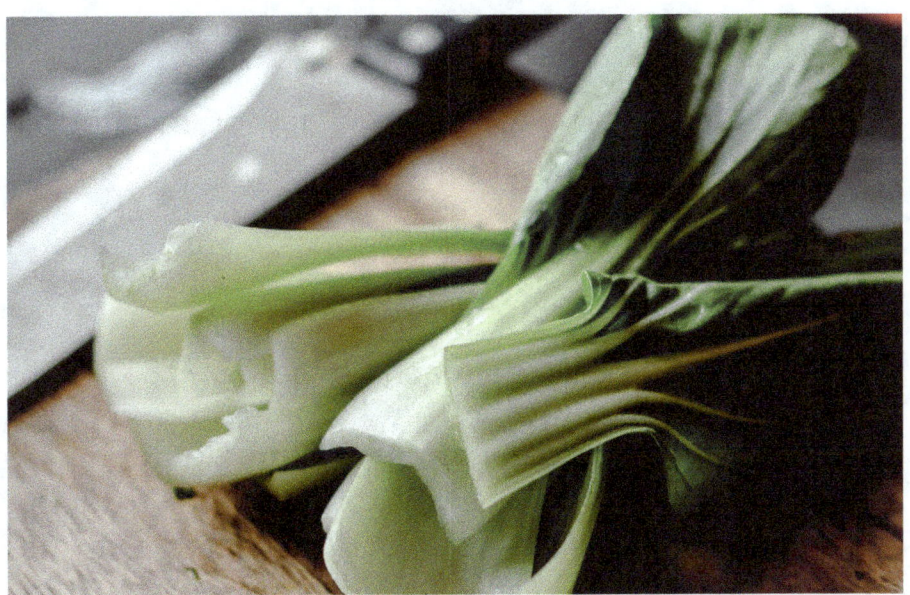

39. ROSEMARY AND GARLIC POTATOES

Cal.: 65 | Fat: 5g | Protein: 11g

Preparation Time: 6 minutes
Cooking Time: 60 minutes
Servings: 4

Ingredients

8 to 10 red-skinned new potatoes, scrubbed, rinsed, and quartered
Olive oil
Coarse salt
Freshly ground black pepper
Garlic powder
2 tsp. fresh rosemary, finely minced
1 tbsp. olive oil
1 tbsp. rendered bacon or duck fat, or unsalted butter (optional)

Directions

1. Preheat the Sous Vide machine to 183°F/83.9°C.

2. Place the potatoes in a bowl and drizzle them with a little olive oil, just enough to coat them. Toss the potatoes to ensure every part is coated with oil.

Season with the 2 tsp. Rosemary, salt, pepper and garlic powder to taste. Toss the potatoes again.

3. Place the butter or bacon or duck fat with the potatoes in a ziploc bag and seal it.

4. Place the bag in your preheated water and set the timer for 1 hour.

5. Place the cooked potatoes in a bowl or on a plate.

6. Serve immediately.

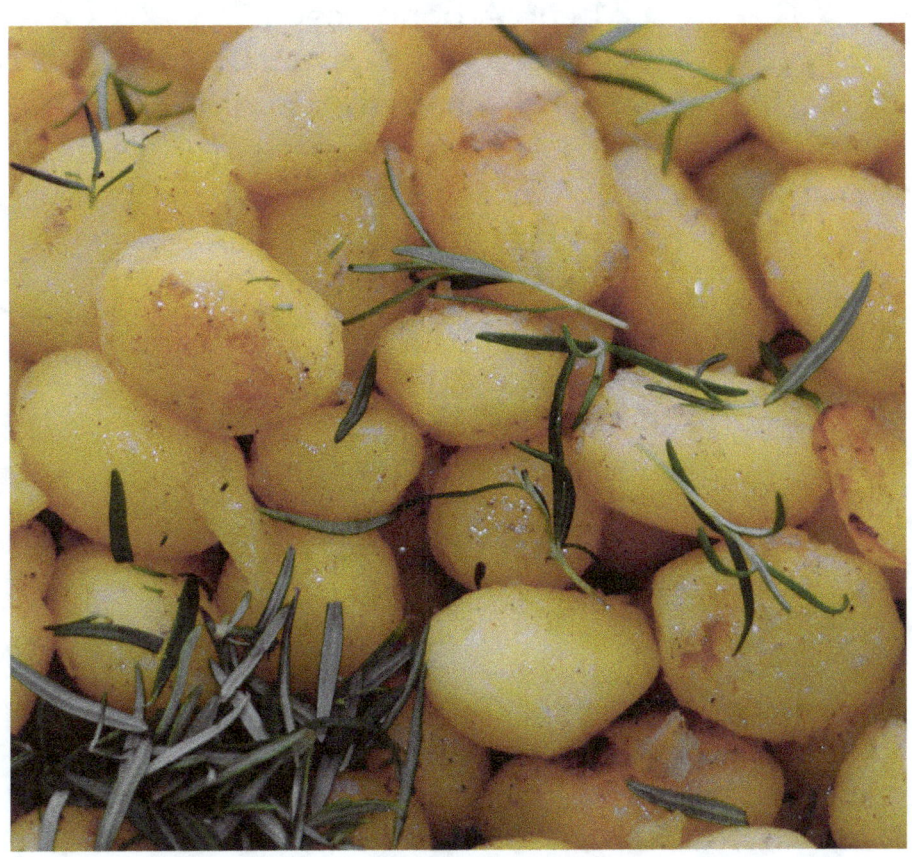

40. TURKEY AND MUSHROOM RISOTTO

Cal.: 129 | Fat: 13g | Protein: 5g

Preparation Time: 6 minutes
Cooking Time: 60 minutes
Servings: 4

Ingredients

1 cup Arborio rice
1 tsp. extra virgin olive oil
1 small yellow onion, peeled and diced
8 to 10 crimini mushrooms, wiped clean and sliced
8 oz. cooked turkey or chicken, diced (leftovers work well!)
2 tbsp. roasted minced garlic (jarred)
720 ml turkey or chicken broth
1 sprig fresh rosemary, leaves only, minced
Salt and pepper to taste
1/3 cup grated Romano cheese

Directions

1. Preheat the Sous Vide machine to 183°F/83°C.

2. Heat up the olive oil in a frying pan on medium heat. Cook the onion and mushrooms until they become tender, about 5 min.

3. Place the first 9 ingredients in the bag you're going to use to sous.

4. Place the bag in your preheated water and set the timer for 1 hour.

5. Place the cooked risotto in 4 bowls and fluff it with a fork.

6. Mix in the cheese and serve.

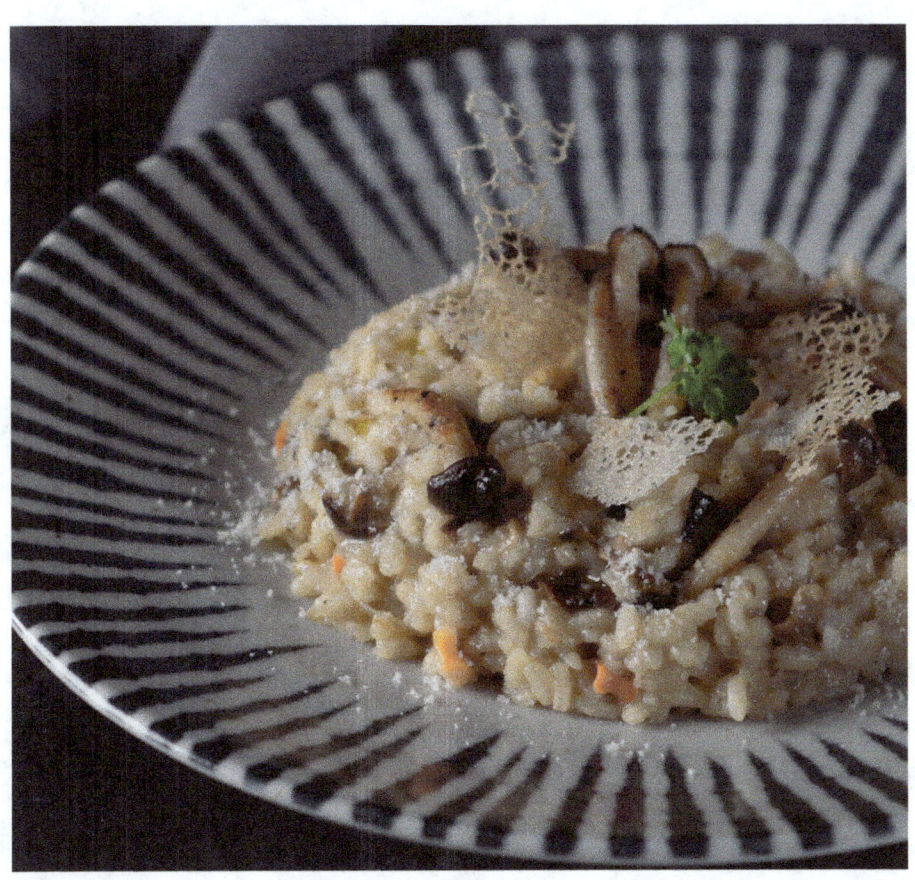

41. EASY FLAVOR-PACKED PICKLES

Cal.: 475 | Fat: 27.8g | Protein: 4.7g

Preparation Time: 11 minutes
Cooking Time: 2 hours 30 minutes
Servings: 10

Ingredients

20 small cucumbers, stems removed
4 medium mason jars
20 black peppercorns
4 garlic cloves, smashed
4 teaspoons fresh dill
For the Pickling Brine:
2-½ cups white wine vinegar
2-½ cups water
½ cup sugar, granulated
2 tablespoons pickling salt

Directions

1. Preheat the water bath to 140°F/60°C.

2. Whisk brine ingredients together in a large mixing bowl until well-combined.

3. Place 5 cucumbers, 5 peppercorns, 1 garlic clove

and 1 teaspoon dill in each Mason jar.

4. Fill each jar with brine and seal the lid tight.

5. Immerse mason jars in the water bath and cook for 2 hours 30 minutes.

6. Remove from the water bath and allow to cool to room temperature.

7. Refrigerate overnight or up to 3 days to brine.

8. Serve with your favorite meals or as a delicious snack.

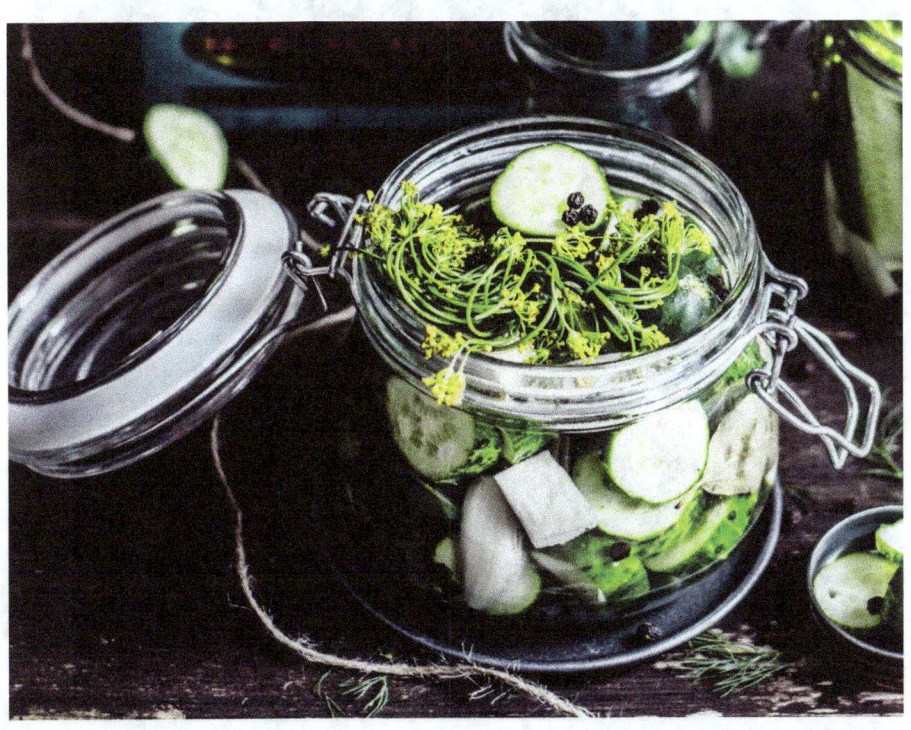

42. CARROT AND CORIANDER SOUP

Cal.: 260 | Fat: 27g | Protein: 12g

Preparation Time: 13 minutes
Cooking Time: 1 hour 45 minutes
Servings: 4

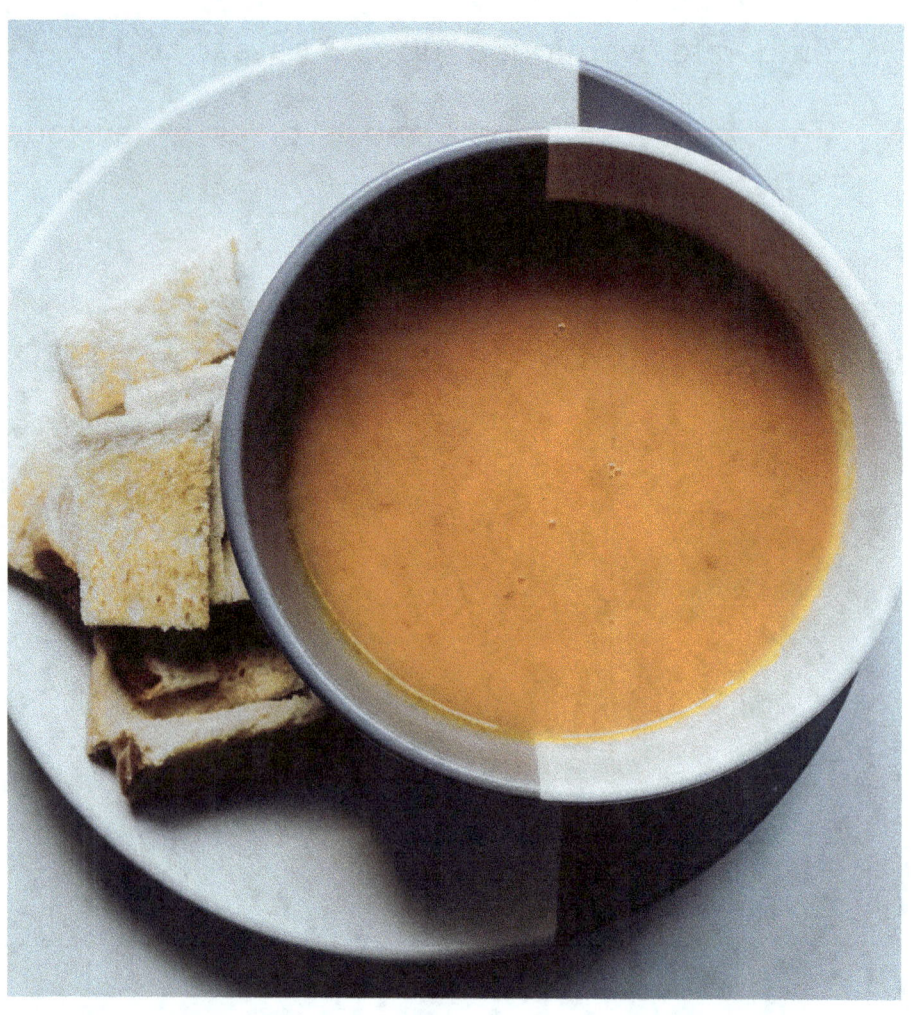

Ingredients

1 lb. carrots
1 cup coconut cream
2 teaspoons ground coriander
1 teaspoon ground cumin
1 garlic clove, crushed
Fresh coriander, chopped, to serve

Directions

1. Set your Sous Vide machine to 190°F/88°C.

2. Put carrots, coconut cream, coriander, cumin and garlic into a Ziploc or vacuum-seal bag and remove all the air. Seal and immerse the bag in the water bath and cook for 1 hour and 45 minutes.

3. Transfer the ingredients to a blender, breaking up the carrots as you remove them, and blend until smooth.

4. Serve warm, topping with chopped coriander to taste.

43. SPICY KOREAN PORK RIBS

Cal.: 536 | Fat: 14.3g | Protein: 89.7g

Preparation Time: 11 minutes
Cooking Time: 2 hours 12 hours
Servings: 4

Ingredients

3 pounds baby back pork ribs, separated into individual ribs
½ cup gochujang
2 tablespoons dark brown sugar
2 tablespoons soy sauce
2 tablespoons rice vinegar
2 teaspoons toasted sesame oil
Salt to taste

Directions

1. Set your Sous Vide Machine to 165°F/74°C.

2. In a bowl, combine the gochujang, brown sugar, soy sauce, vinegar and sesame oil.

3. Season the ribs with salt and place in a vacuum-sealed bag. Add the marinade to the bag and seal.

4. Immerse the bag in the water bath and cook for 12

hours.

5. When the ribs are nearly finished, heat your oven to 450°F/230°C.

6. Remove the ribs from the bag and reserve the marinade. Place the ribs on a baking sheet and brush with the reserved marinade.

7. Cook in the oven for 15 minutes and baste again with marinade. Cook for an additional 10 minutes.

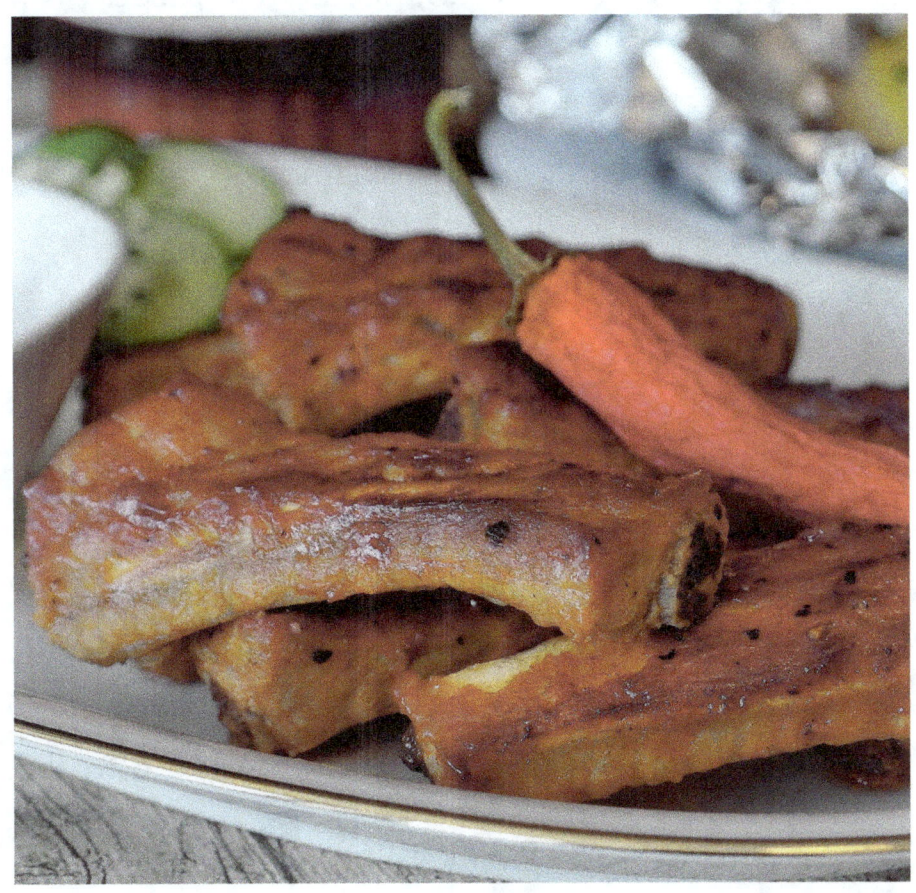

44. APPLE AND CINNAMON PIE

Cal.: 272 | Fat: 3g | Protein: 16g

Preparation Time: 11 minutes
Cooking Time: 2 hours 20 minutes
Servings: 4

Ingredients

2 pounds green, cored, peeled and sliced
3/4 cup sugar
2 tbsp. cornstarch
2 tbsp. butter
2 tsp. ground cinnamon
1 pack puff pastry
2 tbsp. milk
2 tbsp. sugar

Directions

1. Preheat the Sous Vide machine to 160°F/71°C.

2. Put the sliced apples, cornstarch, sugar, cinnamon and butter in the vacuum bag and set the cooking time for 1 hour 30 minutes.

3. When the time is up, cool down the filling to the room temperature.

4. In the meantime, preheat the oven to 375 °F, grease a baking pan, and roll out 1 sheet of the pastry.

5. Pour the filling over the sheet, and cover it with another sheet, seal the sheets on the edges with your fingers.

6. Bake in the preheated oven for 35 minutes.

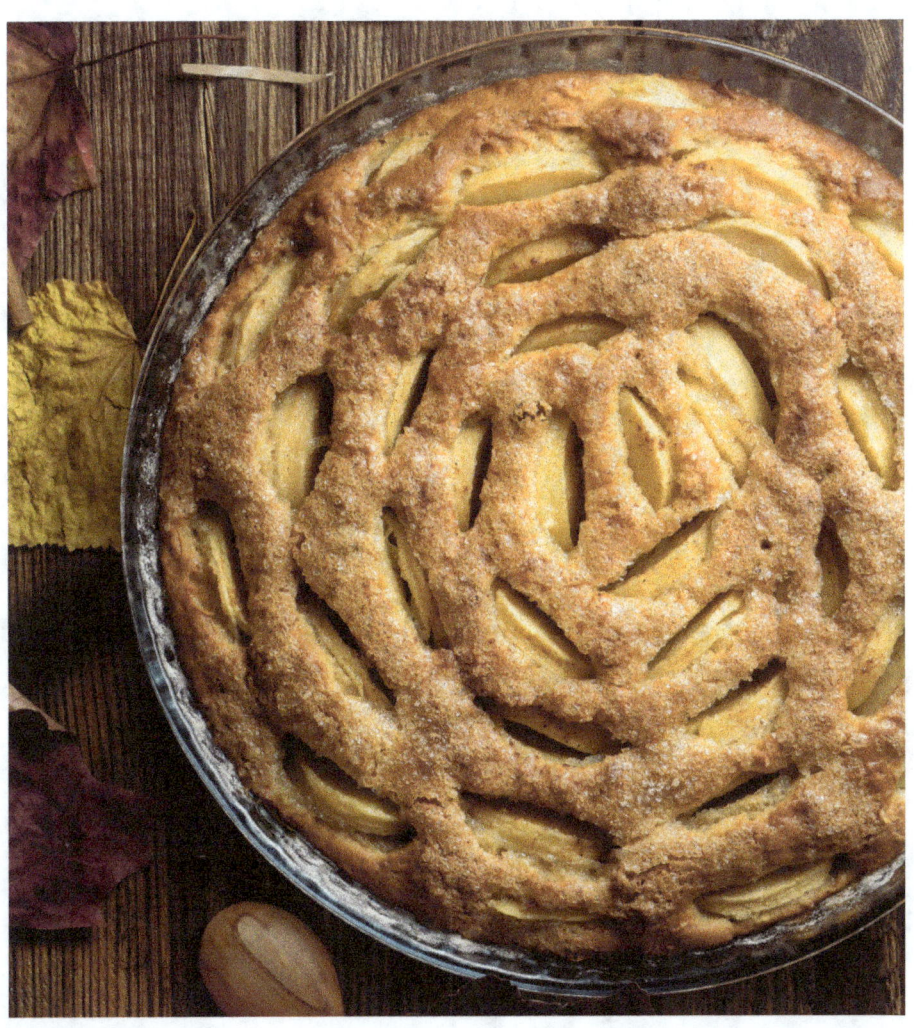

45. DOLCE DE LECHE

Cal.: 91 | Fat: 2.5g | Protein: 2.2g

Preparation Time: 6 minutes
Cooking Time: 2 hours 13 hours
Servings: 8

Ingredients

12 oz. sweetened condensed milk

Directions

1. Preheat your Sous Vide Machine to 185°F/85°C.

2. Put the milk in a bag or a pint size mason jar.

3. Put the bag or Mason jar in your preheated container and set your timer for 13 hours.

4. When the dolce de Leche is cooked, pour it into 4 bowls to serve.

46. WINE AND CINNAMON POACHED PEARS

Cal.: 173 | Fat: 1g | Protein: 0.4g

Preparation Time: 9 minutes
Cooking Time: 2 hours 90 minutes
Servings: 4

Ingredients

4 pears, peeled
2 cinnamon sticks
2 cups red wine
1/3 cup sugar
3-star anise

Directions

1. Preheat the Sous Vide machine to 175°F/79°C. Combine the pears, wine, anise, sugar and cinnamon in a Ziploc bag. Seal and immerse in the preheated water. Cook for 1 hour. Serve the pears drizzle with the wine sauce.

47. OYSTER STEW

Cal.: 376 | Fat: 26g | Protein: 12g

Preparation Time: 9 minutes
Cooking Time: 62 minutes
Servings: 4

Ingredients

4 tablespoons unsalted butter
1 cup thinly sliced leeks
1 small garlic clove, minced
2 cups shucked oysters with liquid
2 cups whole milk
2 cups heavy cream
1 bay leaf
Kosher salt and freshly ground black pepper

Directions

1. Preheat the Sous Vide machine to 120°F/49°C.

2. Melt the butter in a large skillet over medium heat and then add the leeks and garlic. Sauté while stirring until the vegetables are tender. Set aside to cool.

3. In a large ziplock or vacuum-seal bag, combine the oysters, milk, cream, bay leaf, and leek mixture.

Seal the bag using the water displacement method or a vacuum-sealed and then place in the water bath. Set the timer for 1 hour.

4. When the timer goes off, remove the bag from the water bath. Divide the stew into bowls and remove the bay leaf. Season with salt and pepper to taste and serve.

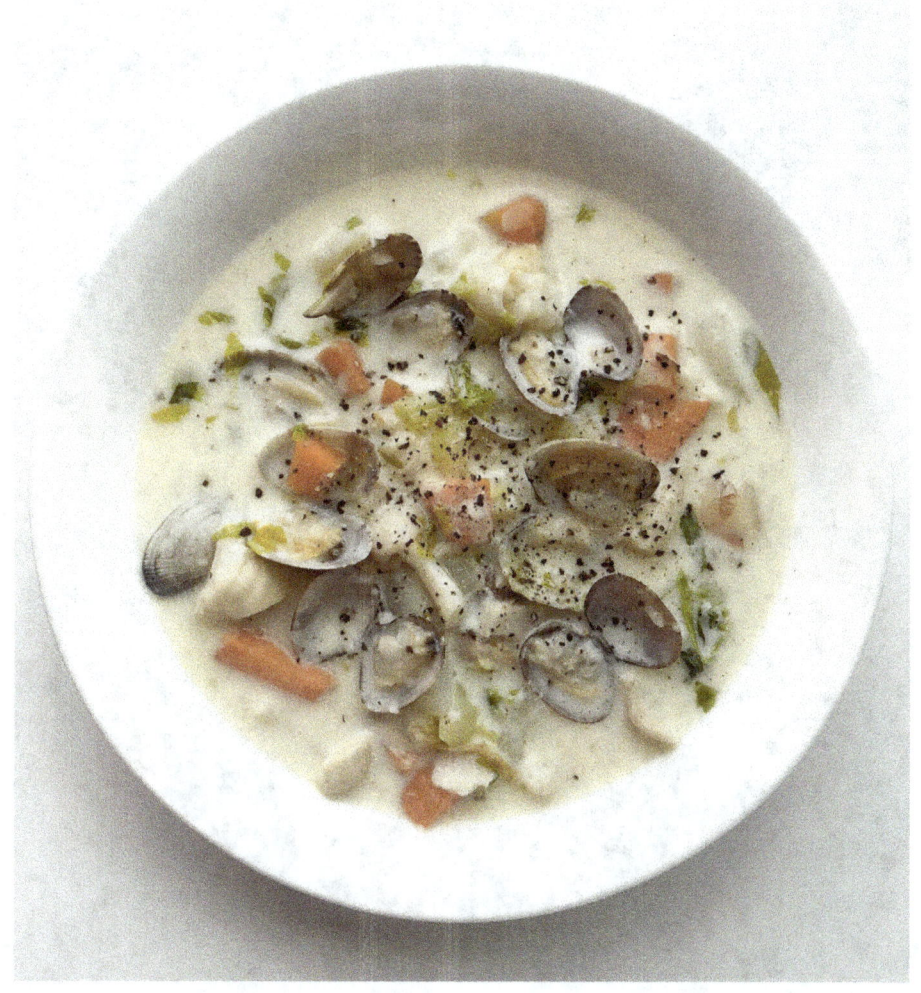

48. BALSAMIC MUSHROOMS AND MIXED HERBS

Cal.: 405 | Fat: 18g | Protein: 12g

Preparation Time: 15 minutes
Cooking Time: 1 hour 60 minutes
Servings: 4

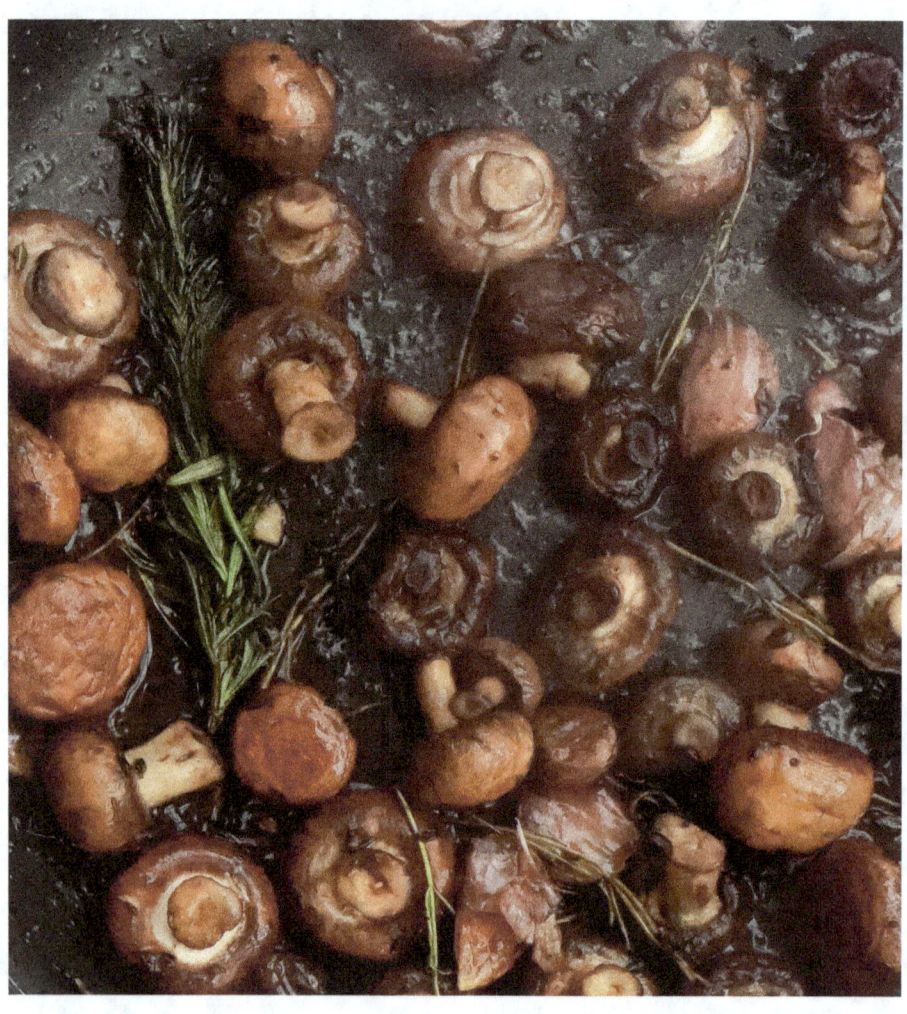

Ingredients

1 pound cremini mushrooms, stems removed
1 tablespoon extra-virgin olive oil
1 tablespoon apple balsamic vinegar
1 teaspoon black pepper, freshly ground
1 teaspoon fresh thyme, minced
1 garlic clove, minced
1 teaspoon kosher salt

Directions

1. Pre-heat your water bath by submerging the immersion circulator and set the temperature at 140°F/60°C.

2. Add all the listed ingredients into a heavy-duty resealable zip bag.

3. Seal bag using the immersion method, Immerse it.

4. Cook for 1 hour.

5. Serve and enjoy!

49. STRACCIATELLA ALLA ROMANA SOUP

Cal.: 391 | Fat: 36g | Protein: 14g

Preparation Time: 11 minutes
Cooking Time: 6 hours
Servings: 8

Ingredients

1 (4-pound whole chicken, trussed
6 cups water
2 cups diced carrots
2 cups diced celery
2 cups diced white onion
Kosher salt and freshly ground black pepper
½ cup grated Parmesan cheese
4 large eggs, beaten
1/4 cup thinly sliced scallion
2 tablespoons freshly squeezed lemon juice
2 tablespoons minced fresh parsley
2 cups baby spinach

Directions

1. Preheat the Sous Vide machine to 150°F/65°C.

2. In a Ziploc or vacuum-seal bag, combine the

chicken, water, carrots, celery and onion. Season with salt and pepper. Seal the bag using the water displacement technique and then place the bag into the hot water bath. Set a timer for 6 hours. Cover the water bath with plastic wrap to minimize water evaporation. Continuously top off the pot with water to keep the chicken fully immersed.

3. When the timer goes off, remove the bag from the water bath and carefully remove the chicken from the bag. Strain the cooking liquid through a fine-mesh strainer into a stockpot. Discard the rest of the ingredients.

4. Let the chicken rest for about 20 minutes or until cool to the touch. Remove and shred the meat.

5. Bring the cooking liquid to a simmer over medium-high heat.

6. In a medium bowl, whisk together the Parmesan, eggs, scallion, lemon juice and parsley. While stirring the stock, slowly pour in the egg mixture in a thin ribbon. Let the eggs cook undisturbed for 1 minute, and then stir.

7. Add the spinach and shredded chicken and simmer until heated through and the spinach has wilted. Season and serve.

50. CARAMELIZED YOGURT WITH GRILLED BERRIES

Cal.: 101 | Fat: 3.5g | Protein: 5.4g

Preparation Time: 60 minutes
Cooking Time: 12 hours
Servings: 8

Ingredients

1 lb. natural yogurt plus 3.5 oz. natural yogurt
12 oz. blueberries
12 oz. raspberries
Mint for garnish

Directions

1. Preheat your Sous Vide Machine to 162°F/72°C.

2. Place the yogurt in a bag and place the bag in the preheated container and set your timer for 12 hours.

3. When nearly finished cooking, prepare an ice bath.

4. Once cooked, place the bag in a bowl, and put the bowl in the ice bath. Allow the yogurt to cool.

5. Open the bag and pour the yogurt into a colander

or sieve that's lined with the muslin cloth. Position the sieve over a bowl and let strain for about an hour.

6. Slowly whisk in the 3.5 ounces of yogurt. Grill the berries on a very hot grill for a short time or heat with a kitchen torch. Garnish with mint to serve.

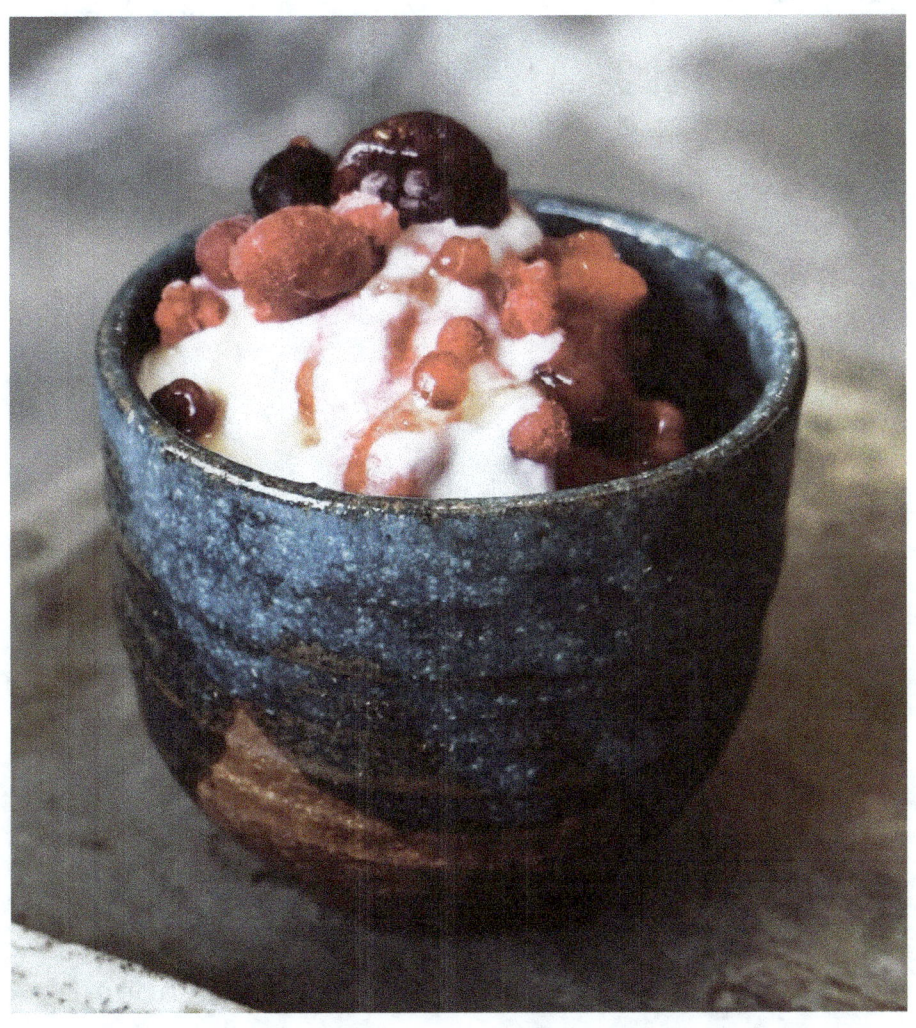

TEMPERATURE CHARTS

🥩 MEAT	°F🌡 TEMPERATURE	⏱ TIME
Beef Steak, rare	129 °F	1 hour 30 min.
Beef Steak, medium-rare	136 °F	1 hour 30min.
Beef Steak, well done	158 °F	1 hour 30min.
Beef Roast, rare	133 °F	7 hours
Beef Roast, medium-rare	140 °F	6 hours
Beef Roast, well done	158 °F	5 hours
Beef Tough Cuts, rare	136 °F	24 hours
Beef Tough Cuts, medium-rare	149 °F	16 hours
Beef Tough Cuts, well done	185 °F	8 hours
Lamb Tenderloin, Rib eye, T-bone, Cutlets	134 °F	4 hours
Lamb Roast, Leg	134 °F	10 hours
Lamb Flank Steak, Brisket	134 °F	12 hours
Pork Chop, rare	136 °F	1 hour
Pork Chop, medium-rare	144 °F	1 hour
Pork Chop, well done	158 °F	1 hour
Pork Roast, rare	136 °F	3 hours

🥩 MEAT	°F TEMPERATURE	⏱ TIME
Pork Roast, medium-rare	144 °F	3 hours
Pork Roast, well done	158 °F	3 hours
Pork Tough Cuts, rare	144 °F	16 hours
Pork Tough Cuts, medium-rare	154 °F	12 hours
Pork Tough Cuts, well done	154 °F	8 hours
Pork Tenderloin	134 °F	1 hour 30min
Pork Baby Back Ribs	165 °F	6 hours
Pork Cutlets	134 °F	5 hours
Pork Spare Ribs	160 °F	12 hours
Pork Belly (quick)	185 °F	5 hours
Pork Belly (slow)	167 °F	24 hours

🐟 FISH AND SEAFOOD	°F TEMPERATURE	⏱ TIME
Fish, tender	104 °F	40 min.
Fish, tender and flaky	122 °F	40 min.
Fish, well done	140 °F	40 min.
Salmon, Tuna, Trout, Mackerel, Halibut, Snapper, Sole	126 °F	30 min.
Lobster	140 °F	50 min.
Scallops	140 °F	50 min.
Shrimp	140 °F	35 min.

🍗 POULTRY	°F 🌡 TEMPERATURE	⏱ TIME
Chicken White Meat, super-supple	140 °F	2 hours
Chicken White Meat, tender and juicy	149 °F	1 hour
Chicken White Meat, well done	167 °F	1 hour
Chicken Breast, bone-in	146 °F	2 hours 30 min.
Chicken Breast, boneless	146 °F	1 hour
Turkey Breast, bone-in	146 °F	4 hours
Turkey Breast, boneless	146 °F	2 hours 30 min.
Duck Breast	134 °F	1 hour 30 min.
Chicken Dark Meat, tender	149 °F	1 hour 30 min.
Chicken Dark Meat, falling off the bone	167 °F	1 hour 30 min.
Chicken Leg or Thigh, bone-in	165 °F	4 hours
Chicken Thigh, boneless	165 °F	1 hour
Turkey Leg or Thigh	165 °F	2 hours
Duck Leg	165 °F	8 hours
Split Game Hen	150 °F	6 hours

🥕 VEGETABLES	°F TEMPERATURE	⏱ TIME
Vegetables, root (carrots, potato, parsnips, beets, celery root, turnips)	183 °F	3 hours
Vegetables, tender (asparagus, broccoli, cauliflower, fennel, onions, pumpkin, eggplant, green beans, corn)	183 °F	1 hour
Vegetables, greens (kale, spinach, collard greens, Swiss chard)	183 °F	3 min.

🍐 FRUITS	°F TEMPERATURE	⏱ TIME
Fruit, firm (apple, pear)	183 °F	45 min.
Fruit, for purée	185 °F	30 min.
Fruit, berries for topping desserts (blueberries, blackberries, raspberries, strawberries, cranberries)	154 °F	30 min.

WHAT TEMPERATURE SHOULD BE USED?

The rule of thumb is that the thicker the piece, the longer it should cook. Higher temperatures shorten the cooking time. Lower temperatures may take longer.

	TEMPERATURE	MIN COOKING TIME	MAX COOKING TIME
EGGS			
Soft Yolk	140°F (60°C)	1 hour	1 hour
Creamy Yolk	145°F (63°C)	¾ hour	1 hour
GREEN VEGETABLES			
Rare	183°F (84°C)	¼ hour	¾ hour
ROOTS			
Rare	183°F (84°C)	1 hour	3 hours
FRUITS			
Warm	154°F (68°C)	1¾ hour	2½ hour
Soft Fruits	185°F (85°C)	½ hour	1½ hour

	TEMPERATURE	MIN COOKING TIME	MAX COOKING TIME
CHICKEN			
Rare	140°F (60°C)	1 hour	3 hours
Medium	150°F (65°C)	1 hour	3 hours
Well Done	167°F (75°C)	1 hour	3 hours
BEEF STEAK			
Rare	130°F (54°C)	1½ hours	3 hours
Medium	140°F (60°C)	1½ hours	3 hours
Well Done	145°F (63°C)	1½ hours	3 hours
ROAST BEEF			
Rare	133°F (54°C)	7 hours	16 hours
Medium	140°F (60°C)	6 hours	14 hours
Well Done	158°F (70°C)	5 hours	11 hours
PORK CHOP BONE-IN			
Rare	136°F (58°C)	1 hour	4 hours
Medium	144°F (62°C)	1 hour	4 hours
Well Done	158°F (70°C)	1 hour	4 hours
PORK LOIN			
Rare	136°F (58°C)	3 hours	5½ hours
Medium	144°F (62°C)	3 hours	5 hours
Well Done	158°F (70°C)	3 hours	3½ hours
FISH			
Tender	104°F (40°C)	½ hour	½ hour
Medium	124°F (51°C)	½ hour	1 hour
Well Done	131°F (55°C)	½ hour	1½ hours

COOKING CONVERSION

TEMPERATURE CONVERSIONS	
CELSIUS	**FAHRENHEIT**
54.5°C	130°F
60.0°C	140°F
65.5°C	150°F
71.1°C	160°F
76.6°C	170°F
82.2°C	180°F
87.8°C	190°F
93.3°C	200°F
100°C	212°F

WEIGHT COVERSION	
½ oz.	15g
1 oz.	30g
2 oz.	60g
3 oz.	85g
4 oz.	110g
5 oz.	140g
6 oz.	170g
7 oz.	200g
8 oz.	225g
9 oz.	255g
10 oz.	280g
11 oz.	310g
12 oz.	340g
13 oz.	370g
14 oz.	400g
15 oz.	425g
1 lb.	450g

LIQUID VOLUME CONVERSION		
CUPS / TABLESPOONS	FL. OUNCES	MILLILITERS
1 cup	8 fl. Oz.	240 ml
¾ cup	6 fl. Oz.	180 ml
2/3 cup	5 fl. Oz.	150 ml
½ cup	4 fl. Oz.	120 ml
1/3 cup	2 ½ fl. Oz.	75 ml
¼ cup	2 fl. Oz.	60 ml
1/8 cup	1 fl. Oz.	30 ml
1 tablespoon	½ fl. Oz.	15 ml

TEASPOON (tsp.) / TABLESPOON (Tbsp.)	MILLILITERS
1 tsp.	5ml
2 tsp.	10ml
1 Tbsp.	15ml
2 Tbsp.	30ml
3 Tbsp.	45ml
4 Tbsp.	60ml
5 Tbsp.	75ml
6 Tbsp.	90ml
7 Tbsp.	105ml

LIQUID VOLUME MEASUREMENTS			
TABLE-SPOONS	TEASPOONS	FLUID OUNCES	CUPS
16	48	8 fl. Oz.	1
12	36	6 fl. Oz.	¾
8	24	4 fl. Oz.	½
5 ½	16	2 2/3 fl. Oz.	1/3
4	12	2 fl. Oz.	¼
1	3	0.5 fl. Oz.	1/16

RECIPE INDEX

Agnolotti with Artichoke Sauce 36
Apple and Cinnamon Pie 96
Asian Inspired Bok Choy 84
Baba Ganoush 22
Bacon Asparagus 21
Balsamic Beets 40
Balsamic Mushrooms and Mixed Herbs 102
Béarnaise Sauce 24
Boneless Strip Steak 72
Brioche and Eggs 26
Caramelized Yogurt with Grilled Berries 106
Carrot and Coriander Soup 92
Cauliflower Alfredo 42
Chicken Marsala 44
Citrus Confit 82
Cured Salmon 30
Dolce De Leche 98
Easy Flavor-Packed Pickles 90
Eggs Benedict 16
Five Spice Pork 46
Frittata with Asparagus 38
Garlic and Rosemary 56
Garlic Broccoli 34
Green Soup 74

Hokkaido Pumpkin	20
Honey Ginger Carrots	14
Hummus	12
Lamb Casserole	52
Lobster Tail with Chimichurri Butter	80
Mahi-Mahi Tacos	66
Overnight Oatmeal with Stewed Fruit Compote	28
Oyster Stew	100
Pears in Pomegranate Juice	32
Poached Halibut	68
Pumpkin Pie	76
Ratatouille	18
Rich and Creamy Polenta	64
Rich and Tasty Duck à Orange	50
Rosemary and Garlic Potatoes	86
Salmon Cakes	60
Salmon with Hollandaise Sauce	78
Shrimp Cocktail	70
Smoked Brisket	48
Spicy Korean Pork Ribs	94
Stracciatella alla Romana Soup	104
Sweet and Spicy Pork Ribs	62
Toast with Flawlessly	58
Turkey and Mushroom Risotto	88
Wine and Cinnamon Poached Pears	99
Yummy Steak Fries	54

www.ingramcontent.com/pod-product-compliance
Lightning Source LLC
Chambersburg PA
CBHW070922080526
44589CB00013B/1406